D1326955

ZERO

Leabharlanna Poiblí Chathair Baile Átha Cliath
Dublin City Public Libraries

JEREMY HUNT

ZERO

Eliminating unnecessary deaths in a post-pandemic NHS

Swift

SWIFT PRESS

First published in Great Britain by Swift Press 2022

1 3 5 7 9 8 6 4 2

Copyright © Jeremy Hunt 2022

The right of Jeremy Hunt to be identified as the Author of this Work has been
asserted in accordance with the Copyright, Designs and Patents Act 1988

Text design and typesetting by Tetragon, London
Printed and bound in Great Britain by CPI Group (UK) Ltd, Croydon, CR0 4YY

A CIP catalogue record for this book is available from the British Library

ISBN: 9781800751224
eISBN: 9781800751231

The names of some individuals in the book have been
changed to preserve their anonymity.

This book is dedicated to the doctors, nurses and managers around the world who have been troubled for too long by the high levels of avoidable harm and death in modern health-care. It is dedicated to the bereaved families who have taken up the cause on behalf of a lost loved one, not for financial gain but simply to try to prevent the same tragedies being repeated. And it is dedicated to the NHS, whose founding values are based on the principle that every single patient matters.

All royalties from this book will be donated to Patient Safety Watch, which funds research by Imperial College London into preventable harm and death.

CONTENTS

INTRODUCTION

Could this be a 1948 moment?

1948 was the year a Labour government, with cross-party support, set up the National Health Service. Health Minister Aneurin Bevan famously dealt with opposition from the doctors' union, the BMA, by 'stuff[ing] their mouths with gold'.[1] He had opposition from Conservatives in parliament who, while supporting the principle, wanted GPs to be employees of the new service but keep hospitals independent (Bevan's plan did the opposite). To his credit, he was willing to smash whatever china necessary to get the NHS off the ground – and in the process created what has become our most treasured national institution, described in poll after poll as the single biggest reason people are proud to be British.[2]

The NHS has stood the test of time because the values it stands for have become entwined with what it means to be British. We are proud that whoever and wherever you are – rich or poor, young or old, north or south – you can always get the healthcare you need, irrespective of the size of your bank balance. We were not actually the first country to set up a universal healthcare system (that honour goes to New Zealand[3]), but we are the probably the best known. By setting up the NHS at a pivotal moment for the world, right after the Second World War, we helped make universal provision part of the definition of a civilised country. Forty-three countries now offer a comprehensive version of it, including most developed countries, except of course

America. Most others are planning universal provision. The NHS has had a huge influence beyond its shores.

But today, that pride in the NHS is starkly at odds with the exhausting daily reality for doctors and nurses. As the service starts its slow, blinking recovery from the Covid-19 pandemic, many feel a sense of helplessness. Frontline professionals are experiencing 'burnout' in record numbers.[4] Patients are wearily coming to terms with huge backlogs that have built up for cancer care or elective surgery. The institution is crying out for renewal, not just because of the threat of new viruses but because of the changing nature of illness caused by an ageing population.

In this book, I argue that the foundation of any reforms must be to improve the quality as well as the quantity of care delivered. NHS care, for all the pride we feel in it, is not always the best. In most studies, the NHS is around the middle of the pack for the quality of care it offers, tending to do better on the accessibility of care than outcomes.[5] But why shouldn't NHS care be of the highest quality too?

Right now, that seems a tall order. Enormous backlogs in treatment have built up during the pandemic. If they are not managed properly, there will be pressure to compromise on standards of safety, which will reduce, rather than increase, the quality of NHS care. Some go further and say the NHS can *never* be the highest quality, for financial reasons: a taxpayer-funded system will never be able to afford the billions needed to pay for advances in modern medicine. Others think there is an inevitable trade-off between access and quality: 'free' systems will never be able to match the standards of care in private ones, because they lack the incentive to put customers first.

Having been Health Secretary for longer than anyone else – with all the ups and downs that involved – I profoundly disagree. The pandemic showed the brilliance of British science and the dedication of the

NHS workforce, so two key foundations are in place. Funding matters, although, as I will discuss later, the relationship between quality and money is more complicated than first meets the eye. But to offer the very best care we need to address a major structural problem, one that is faced not just by the NHS but by countries everywhere: finding a way to deal more honestly and humanely with the shockingly high levels of avoidable harm and death in modern healthcare systems.

Most tragedies are treated as 'inevitable', when in fact they could be prevented simply and cheaply. According to the WHO there are 2.6 million avoidable deaths every year in healthcare systems, making it a global top ten killer, affecting more people than tuberculosis or malaria, and nearly as many as HIV and road traffic accidents.[6] We need to become better at learning from mistakes.

Other industries have succeeded in tackling avoidable harm and death through a root-and-branch change in culture. As Health Secretary, I initially shied away from 'culture change' as being too nebulous and unlikely to have any practical impact. Ultimately, however, I concluded it was the most important change of all, without which improvements only have limited impact at best. Change is hard to deliver, but surely our forebears were no less weary – or broke – recovering from the Second World War in 1948? Focusing on delivering the safest, highest quality care in a way that eliminates avoidable harm and tragedy is the way to set the NHS up for the rest of the century – our very own 1948 moment.

This book is not about me, but I should briefly explain how my interest in eliminating harm in modern healthcare systems arose. My journey started on Monday, 3 September 2012.

It was a glorious late summer day. As the government minister responsible for putting on the London 2012 Olympic Games, I was at the gleaming new Stratford stadium for the Paralympics. Despite the excitement of the sport, I was rather preoccupied. The Prime Minister, David Cameron, had come back from his holiday and was starting a process that always terrifies even hardened ministers: a Cabinet reshuffle.

I had no idea what was in store for me. Lots of pundits thought I would be sacked. Although I had just helped deliver a successful Olympics, I had been embroiled in the Leveson Inquiry into Rupert Murdoch's BSkyB bid. My special adviser had been forced to quit, and for days I had woken up with journalists waiting outside my front door wanting the 'money shot' of me leaving home on the day I resigned. Although the Leveson Inquiry eventually vindicated me,[7] there were many wild accusations flying around – the *Guardian* even printed a huge, grainy picture of me on their front page with the headline 'Minister for Murdoch'.[8] As I sat in the Olympic Stadium, amidst the cheers and excitement of the athletics, I felt anxious awaiting the Prime Minister's call. I knew I was vulnerable.

The next morning the summons to No. 10 came. As I walked through the famous black door, I experienced the well-oiled chore-ography of British government reshuffles. Ministers are met as soon as they've crossed the threshold into No. 10 and discreetly shown to a waiting room – always avoiding other Cabinet ministers on their way in or out. I was shown to the White Room, a beautiful room on the first floor used for bilateral meetings with visiting heads of government. Then there was a knock on the door, and I was ushered down to the Cabinet Room. On one side of the long, oval-shaped table sat just two people: the Prime Minister and his trusted chief of staff Ed Llewellyn. I sat directly opposite them nervously.

Then I got the shock of my life. Cameron asked me to be Health Secretary. For someone who had been under the cosh, it was a huge promotion.

He was in transmit mode, so didn't pause for breath as he started outlining what he wanted me to do with the job. 'We need someone in this job who speaks English' was one of the phrases he used alluding to the difficulties the government had experienced in communicating Andrew Lansley's reforms. Then he suddenly stopped in mid flow and said, 'First, I should check – will you accept the job?'

'You bet,' I said, 'even though I am pretty daunted.' Quite the understatement.

After all, this wasn't just any department. This was the department that oversaw our most treasured institution and the fifth biggest employer in the world.[9] Uniquely, 80% of health funding in the UK comes through central taxation,[10] so pretty much everything that goes wrong is laid at the door of politicians. Budget increases would be difficult amid tight national finances. However much money you gave, for many it would never be enough. And any attempt to change our precious institution would spark fierce opposition, as Lansley's 2012 reforms had shown.

But my trepidation at taking up a potentially poisoned chalice was overshadowed by the sense of awe: to be working in a job where your decisions don't just have a long-term impact but make an immediate and life-changing difference to people's lives is unusual in politics. It was a huge responsibility.

As I left Downing Street, I told the media that being responsible for the NHS was the biggest privilege of my life.[11] It was a hurried, made-for-camera comment. But if it was manufactured initially, I soon came to believe it from the bottom of my heart. I had just agreed to something that would change not just my political career but the direction and purpose of my life.

When I accepted the job, I was an outsider to the world of health. But dealing with inexperienced ministers is something civil servants are quite used to, indeed trained for. When I walked to my new office in Richmond House, on the other side of Whitehall from the Downing Street gates, I was met by extremely welcoming officials. They were somewhat battered after the battles they had been fighting over the Health and Social Care Act, but could not have been kinder or more supportive as I got to grips with the immense task at hand.

Unfortunately, I also went on to discover practices in modern medicine that shocked me to the core.

I came to realise this largely by speaking with patients, something I ended up doing in a very direct way because of something that happened at a rather curious moment: Margaret Thatcher's funeral.

Held in St Paul's Cathedral, it was of course no ordinary funeral. As a member of the Cabinet I was sitting in a row behind Gordon Brown, Tony Blair and John Major. I remember singing 'I Vow to Thee My Country' and thinking it must rank as one of the most British moments of my life.

The eulogy was delivered by Richard Chartres, the Bishop of London and a long-standing friend of Margaret Thatcher's. He read out a letter she had received from a nine-year-old boy called David, to which she had replied personally. I sat there, and thought: In my seven months as Health Secretary I haven't read a single letter from an NHS patient. If Margaret Thatcher had found the time to do personal replies as Prime Minister, couldn't I?

Not, of course, that I didn't receive correspondence. The Department of Health received more letters than any other government department. There was an army of fifty officials in the correspondence unit, whose job was to draft replies and to a certain extent protect ministers from the highly personal and emotional missives received from people who had experienced problems with their care. But it felt wrong that I was not actually seeing any letters myself. Good chief executives stay closely in touch with what their customers are saying – and although the NHS is not a business the principle is the same. So when I went back to my office I asked my civil servants to pass on to me one letter every day for a personal reply. I wanted to send a handwritten letter, not just 'top and tail' a letter drafted by officials.

I didn't know it at the time, but this request sent the department into a spin. Sir Humphrey-like meetings were held behind my back to work out if they could dissuade me from such a thoroughly dangerous idea. They saw their job as shielding me from such letters, not exposing me to them. Furthermore, it was the job of hospitals and not the department to deal with 'local complaints'. No letters came forth.

So I chased the department. And about a month later the first letter arrived.

'I am just writing to thank you for the fantastic NHS care I received...'

'No,' I said. The point was not to tell me what was going right, but to show me what was going wrong.

Eventually, I did start getting some proper complaint letters. They were eye-opening and sometimes horrifying. It didn't matter what form they came in – sometimes an email, sometimes shaky handwriting from an older person, sometimes on scraps of notepaper with terrible spelling – the cry for help was clear. Stories about young children lodged particularly in my mind, as a father of three. One of the earlier letters hit me especially hard: it was from a man in Cumbria, writing about his teenage daughter who had killed herself the day after an appointment with a mental health nurse.

In the very first letter I replied to, I apologised for the terrible care someone had received. The next day my letter came back with a note from officials saying, 'Apologies not permitted.' Presumably someone was worried about a legal admission of liability. However, I knew that the law is perfectly sensible in this respect and apologies do not count as an admission of guilt. The letter went out unchanged.

I then got into a daily routine of replying to one such letter every morning. I always asked for the day's letter to be sitting on my desk waiting for me when I arrived for work, with time put aside in the diary to allow me to do a handwritten reply. As it was the first thing I did every day, those letters shaped my day. They also persuaded me of something: I needed to focus my attention on preventable harm and death. Many of the stories in this book come from those letters, although where requested I have changed names to protect anonymity.

Mistakes happen. In most fields the consequences are limited. In healthcare they can be fatal.

Nothing I say about the mistakes I recount in the pages that follow is a reflection on the competence or dedication of NHS professionals. During nearly six years in office, my encounters with the care they provided were always humbling. I remember meeting a nurse who had tracked down the long-lost relatives of a dying man and arranged for him to fly to Ireland to see them for the first time in twenty years; I met a heart surgeon who stopped a human heart in front of my eyes and then restarted it half an hour later when the surgery was complete; I was transfixed by a care home manager whose passion was putting a smile on the faces of residents unable to talk because of late stage dementia; I visited a GP who insisted on washing the body of a dead patient before the undertakers took it away; and I met countless cheerful, hard-working healthcare assistants who taught me to wash beds between patients and grinned when it was my turn to empty a commode.

The problem does not lie with individuals, but with healthcare systems around the world that generally 'go after' someone when something goes wrong, making it impossible for professionals to be open about mistakes. The result is a blame game that stops learning and allows the same mistake to be repeated, often countless times. Ending that culture – and the harm and tragedy associated with it – became my focus. It is why I have written this book.

I saw that flawed culture on a huge scale in the aftermath of the Mid Staffs hospital scandal, a terrible failure of care that led to between 400 and 1,200 unnecessary and often cruel deaths over four years between 2005 and 2009.[12] My predecessor had set up a public inquiry led by Sir Robert Francis, which was due to report early in 2013. Because we knew the report wouldn't pull any punches, the issue hung like a shadow over the Department of Health in my first few months.

'You have to understand that in healthcare we harm ten per cent of patients,' I was told wearily by Sir David Nicholson, who was the chief executive of the NHS from 2006 to 2014. By his own admission, David had made mistakes over Mid Staffs, but I developed enormous respect for him. We had little in common politically, but he was the most effective manager I ever met. By 'harm' he meant damage done to patients because of medical errors – in other words, something that could be avoided.

'If ten per cent of patients are harmed, how many actually *die* as a result?' I asked.

We have more data on this kind of thing than anywhere else in the world, so a remarkably precise answer came back. According to a study led by Helen Hogan and Nick Black, two eminent academics at the London School of Hygiene and Tropical Medicine, around 4% of hospital deaths had a 50% or more chance of being avoidable.[13] When you do the maths, that turns out to be a rather dry way of saying that there are 150 avoidable deaths every single week. Many of these would have been frail elderly patients with a relatively short time left, but none the less, a huge number of lives were being cut short.

If English rates were typical across the world – and the NHS appears to be about the middle of the pack by international standards – that means millions of deaths a year globally, as indeed the WHO now recognises. But the crucial difference between deaths from medical error and deaths from, say, cancer is that *every single one of them is immediately preventable*. We are not waiting for a miracle cure. They could be stopped right now if best practice was followed.

If my daily letters were the building blocks for a mission, Mid Staffs became the catalyst that galvanised it.

My first instinct was to focus on transparency. All these avoidable deaths felt like a major scandal – but one that no one seemed to know about.

There seemed to be a kind of omertà around avoidable deaths in the NHS. This was partly because people at the top of the service thought their political masters would not want the bad publicity. But it was probably more from an understandable worry that talking about such deaths would damage public confidence in the NHS. Unfortunately, the corrosive consequence of such thinking was all kinds of terrible cover-ups in which both the Department of Health and the NHS were sadly complicit. When problems like Mid Staffs were identified, the default response was to try to sort them out behind closed doors without the public ever finding out.

That approach prevented rapid, decisive action from being taken. Too often managers who had failed were recycled to jobs in a different part of the country where they continued to make the same mistakes. And because of the secrecy, the wheels of change ground very slowly. Failures at Mid Staffs went on for four years before decisive action was taken. In many ways, the scandal was not that terrible things happened, but that they went on for so long before being stopped. But how could there be impetus for change when no one knew that it was needed?

After a lot of resistance from both the Department of Health and the NHS, I introduced a transparent and independent ratings system for hospitals, GP surgeries and care homes – the first healthcare system in the world to do so. Based on the Ofsted system used successfully for schools, it introduced a four-point scale for every organisation. All were graded either 'outstanding', 'good', 'requires improvement' or 'inadequate'. An 'inadequate' rating usually led to the hospital being put into 'special measures' with wholesale management change.

Hospitals are much bigger and more complex organisations than schools, so underneath the overall rating were sub-ratings on safety, outcomes, responsiveness, compassion and leadership. The process of getting to a rating was a huge undertaking, with around fifty inspectors (many of whom were themselves doctors and nurses) descending onto a hospital for three days.[14]

The result was that in the first three years, twenty-eight hospitals were put into special measures.[15] Most had their management changed and the majority then showed improvements. A few took a very long time to turn things around but, four years on, nearly three million more patients were being treated in 'good' or 'outstanding' hospitals.[16]

Had I stopped being Health Secretary after a year or two, I would have probably said that the key to better patient care was that kind of transparency, perhaps accompanied by targeted campaigns in particular areas like medication error or sepsis. But the longer I continued, the more I became convinced there was an even more fundamental issue that needed tackling. In medicine, we are just not as good as we need to be at learning from mistakes and spreading best practice. This was writ large at the start of the Covid-19 pandemic, when Europe and North America failed to learn from the much more successful approach taken in places like Korea and Taiwan[17] – but the issues are the same in more normal times.

So I began to look at how other industries worked, including the airline, nuclear and oil industries. I read books about patient safety like *The Checklist Manifesto* by Atul Gawande, which have saved thousands of lives through systematising changes in behaviour. What I learned was the importance of culture change when it comes to learning from error. If the priority is punishing individuals after a tragedy *pour encourager les autres*, the only real consequence is backside-protecting and cover-ups. If, however, your main focus is preventing tragedies from being repeated, you need exactly the opposite: rapid, no-blame investigations and urgent dissemination of any lessons learned. That can only happen if frontline professionals feel able to speak truthfully and openly when things go wrong, as they inevitably will.

How do you get there? I start this book with a section on the core issues: a pervasive blame culture, staff shortfalls and resourcing. I then go on to look in more detail at what causes that flawed culture: an obsession with targets that can make numbers more important than people; over-rigid hierarchies; fear of litigation; groupthink; and the risk of certain groups being marginalised.

Then I look at the best solutions: restoring the doctor–patient relationship with proper accountability for every single individual in the system; transparency; smart (but not detrimental) use of technology; and prioritising prevention as well as cure. These are big topics in their own right but my focus is on how they can help to prevent avoidable harm and death. I therefore explicitly examine the challenges facing the NHS through a patient safety lens, although fully recognising that there are other equally valid ways of doing so, such as medical advances, new models of care or health inequalities.

Finally, I reflect on the challenge of implementing such solutions in the world's fifth largest bureaucracy, including my own battle with junior doctors and the role patients have to play. I also ask whether it is motivating or demotivating to aim for 'zero harm', given we are unlikely ever to achieve it. In short, I look at how to reduce avoidable harm and death from every possible angle, and try to talk as much about solutions as about the problem.

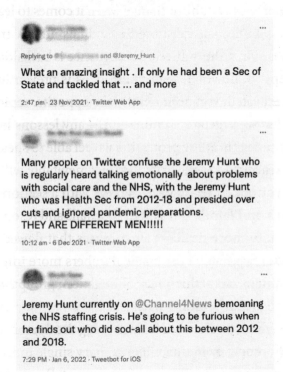

Replying to @██████ and @Jeremy_Hunt

What an amazing insight . If only he had been a Sec of State and tackled that ... and more

2:47 pm · 23 Nov 2021 · Twitter Web App

Many people on Twitter confuse the Jeremy Hunt who is regularly heard talking emotionally about problems with social care and the NHS, with the Jeremy Hunt who was Health Sec from 2012-18 and presided over cuts and ignored pandemic preparations.
THEY ARE DIFFERENT MEN!!!!!

10:12 am · 6 Dec 2021 · Twitter Web App

Jeremy Hunt currently on @Channel4News bemoaning the NHS staffing crisis. He's going to be furious when he finds out who did sod-all about this between 2012 and 2018.

7:29 PM · Jan 6, 2022 · Tweetbot for iOS

This is not a memoir, but, as I examine these issues, I cannot avoid some consideration of my own record. Where I identify a problem, some will understandably criticise the fact I did not solve it despite a long time in the job – as in the tweets above. Inevitably, in a job with such responsibility you don't get everything right, and you learn things as you go along. We should all want our politicians to do that.

Although reflecting on those six years is necessarily a subjective process, I have, none the less, tried to be as objective as I can. That includes successes already mentioned, such as the fact that by the end of my tenure three million more patients were being treated every year in 'good' or 'outstanding' hospitals. It covers failures such as the disappointing progress in recruiting more GPs and the unintended consequences of the junior doctors' strike.

But most of the time the outcomes were somewhere in between – some progress, but much more needing to be done. The best example of this is perhaps maternity safety, where there was a marked reduction in baby deaths[18] – but still levels of harm far higher than in countries like Sweden.[19] Even though some will disagree with my analysis, I make no apology for presenting it: if we want the NHS to be the safest and highest quality healthcare system in the world, we should seek to learn from successes and setbacks in its history.

I wrote this book on the basis of my own experiences, interviewing many patients and families. It is told unashamedly from their point of view. I try to be fair but do not attempt to balance such stories with the alternate viewpoints of the hospitals, surgeries or clinicians with whom they interacted – that is a job for those conducting inquiries or inquests. For that reason I have not identified the names of the hospitals where such events took place unless the issues to which the stories relate are widely in the public domain.

My father worked in NHS management after he retired from his career in the Royal Navy, and my mother was a nurse during the 1950s and 1960s, about the same time as *Call the Midwife*. I have three wonderful children born thanks to the NHS. But perhaps my best experience of NHS compassion came more recently, when my four-year-old daughter fell off a running machine and suffered serious burns on her back.

Being with her at all hours in the burns unit of the Chelsea and Westminster hospital made me appreciate why the NHS is different: it's not that doctors and nurses in other countries aren't equally kind – anyone who goes into medicine chooses to make caring for others central to their life. But unlike other systems, because the NHS does not bill people directly for their care, we are always patients and never customers. That means the compassion you experience is never generated by a financial motive and is always utterly genuine.

I think that is why so many people talk about the quality of NHS care with a certain awe. It is why the British have taken the NHS to their hearts. But with 150 avoidable deaths every week – even outside a pandemic – how often does our system support doctors and nurses to demonstrate the compassion my family experienced – and how often does it frustrate them?

PART ONE

The Three Big Causes of Avoidable Harm

1

Blame

As Health Secretary, perhaps the most difficult meeting I ever had was on 2 March 2015. It was the day before I had to give a statement to parliament on the Kirkup Inquiry into baby deaths at Furness General Hospital, part of Morecambe Bay Trust.[1] The meeting was with a group of families who had lost their babies due to poor care at the hospital. They were angry and wanted justice and closure. What made them most angry was that some of the staff allegedly responsible were still working at the trust. I had a lot of sympathy – but as I dug deeper I came to a rather unexpected conclusion about the motivations of the staff involved, namely that they were more likely to have been scared rather than evil.

Simon Davey and Liza Brady had lost their son Alex, who was still-born. An inquest discovered failings in his care by midwives, who did not involve doctors early enough during Liza's labour.[2] A subsequent report by the Parliamentary and Health Service Ombudsman pointed to the poor supervision of midwives.[3]

Carl Hendrickson lost not just his son Chester, but his wife Nittaya too. She suffered a rare embolism after giving birth to Chester and died within an hour. Chester had brain damage and passed away the next day. Important heart monitor documents were lost, along with other hospital emails. The midwife responsible for the birth had dismissed Nittaya's fits as fainting.

Ahead of the meeting, my staff told me that Carl had brought his eleven-year-old son Conrad with him. I asked them to offer to look after Conrad during the meeting, as it would be likely to cover pretty difficult subject matter. No, the reply came, he insists he wants his son to be with him at the meeting. Carl later told a newspaper that was because he thought, 'You've lost your mum and brother, and when you grow up I want you to know that I took this to the top man in government, and that we asked some awkward questions.'[4]

Awkward questions were exactly what those families asked. How could staff involved in such incidents still be working in the same maternity unit? Why did the trust cover up what had happened for so

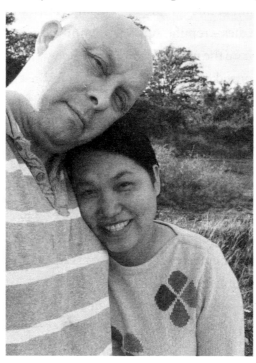

Carl and Nittaya Hendrickson

long? Why did the NHS not launch a proper national inquiry sooner? The sense of injustice was palpable, and I felt deeply ashamed of what had happened to them.

Because they had been forced to fight so hard for the truth, I felt I needed to be totally honest about what I could and could not do. That would include saying things they might not want to hear.

'If this was a dictatorship,' I said, 'and I could stand in parliament tomorrow and say that all the staff involved have been fired forthwith, that might give you satisfaction. But what signal would it send to maternity staff in another hospital, the next time something went wrong? Might they decide the safest thing was for them, too, to cover up their mistakes?'

The covering up of mistakes is endemic. Not just in the NHS, but in most modern healthcare systems. It arises because, in the justified quest for accountability – particularly for something as serious as when a patient dies – reputations, careers and money are at stake. But how do you square the need for accountability with the need for space to learn from mistakes – even the gravest of mistakes, which lead to loss of life? In the end, that is the key to eliminating the 150 avoidable deaths we have every week in England.

So how do you replace a blame culture with a learning culture? In this opening section, I will look at the main causes of avoidable harm and death: a flawed culture, workforce shortages and resources. Because the latter two are discussed and debated endlessly (at least in the UK), I then spend the next section looking in more detail at the root causes of poor culture in healthcare workplaces, before going on to consider solutions.

But first, let's look more carefully at the issue of blame. Why does it get in the way of making improvements that absolutely everyone wants to make?

———

James Titcombe is perhaps the UK's best-known patient safety campaigner, and his focus has always been on getting the culture in healthcare systems right. He differentiates between a 'just culture' and a 'blame culture'. His own life was shattered by the loss of his son, Joshua, after he was born at Furness General Hospital. He wasn't at the March 2015 meeting because we had already met – in fact, he was the person who had persuaded me to set up the Kirkup Inquiry.

The first time I met James, I was struck by his combination of calm modesty and inner steel. He worked as a nuclear industry project manager at Sellafield in Cumbria, and exuded the quiet pragmatism you would expect from someone who knows what it is like to be responsible for life-and-death decisions. But as he sat in the beige armchair in my office and began to tell his story, I could see that alongside that calmness he had extraordinary determination to find out the truth about what happened to his son.[5]

Everything had started with such promise. At around 5 a.m. on an October morning, his wife Hoa's contractions began. The hospital advised him not to bring her in until the contractions got more frequent, which they did – quickly – and by 6.30 a.m. James and Hoa were in the car to Furness General Hospital.

As a project manager, James was a natural planner. So before they left home, he carefully made sure the cot was ready in the house and a car seat for the baby in place. But as he started the engine, he never imagined he wouldn't be bringing his wife home for two weeks – with both their lives irreversibly scarred.

After a short labour, Joshua Titcombe was born at 7.38 a.m. He was blue, floppy and appeared not to be breathing. The midwife took him straightaway to another room for an oxygen blast, after which he let out a loud cry. Everyone relaxed. The new mum and dad had tears of pride in their eyes.

Then Hoa became very ill with a ragingly high temperature. James called for help, and eventually she was given antibiotics and fluids for an infection. James wondered: if she had an infection, did Joshua too? But the midwives dismissed any concerns. The baby was fine. As a layman, the new father accepted their advice. That night, James went home relatively relaxed. Joshua was supposedly fine, and Hoa was getting the treatment she needed.

Later, however, Joshua became visibly ill. He was cold and grunting. At one point, in the middle of the night, he was making such loud noises that Hoa rang the bell by her bed. A midwife came in and took Joshua away for half an hour, before returning and telling Hoa that he was fine.

But the midwife did not consult Joshua's notes, including the yellow observation chart that would have shown his temperature was abnormally low – a classic sign of sepsis.[6] Nor did she consult a doctor. Those temperature charts subsequently went missing – never to be recovered.

The reassurance turned out to be false – and shortly afterwards Joshua deteriorated. James was called back to the hospital. He arrived to find his wife in tears and Joshua being looked at by a doctor in a different room. James got one glimpse of his son before he was told to leave. Standing outside, he saw a team of medics gather round as Joshua was put on a full ventilator, no longer able to breathe with his own lungs.

Surely, James thought, Joshua hadn't collapsed from the same infection as his wife? Not when he'd raised the issue so many times and been reassured to the contrary?

But admitting they had got the diagnosis wrong was too much for the staff, so this time James was told that it looked as if Joshua was suffering from a heart defect. Later, this untruth would be finessed as a 'differential diagnosis', a snap judgement made in the heat of the moment. But James was starting to lose faith in the system.

Finally, Joshua was put on the antibiotics he should have been given at the outset. But it was too late. Joshua had sepsis, just like his mother. If he had been given antibiotics at the same time as her, he would have had a 95% chance of survival. Now it was touch-and-go.

The little baby was rushed to a specialist hospital in Manchester at 11 p.m. He received extremely professional care, and James and Hoa were advised it might be appropriate to put him on an ECMO, a heart and lung machine for babies, which would allow Joshua's heart and lungs time to rest while the doctors reoxygenated his blood artificially.

After careful deliberation, the parents gave permission for Joshua to be flown by helicopter to the Freeman Hospital in Newcastle. Again, the care was excellent. Over the next few days Joshua appeared to make good progress, and the consultant overseeing his care decided

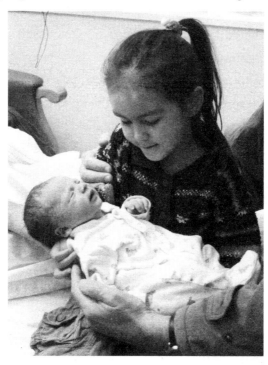

Joshua Titcombe with his sister Emily

to wean him off the ECMO machine. James went to bed that night thinking that the next day Joshua would be breathing with his own lungs. He began to allow himself to imagine bringing his baby home, the car seat ready and the nursery and cot still in place. His parents would be there to welcome the new arrival to the family.

But when James and Hoa went in the next morning, it was clear that something had gone terribly wrong. The weaning process hadn't worked. Worse still, the doctors had discovered that Joshua's lung was more necrotic – rotten – from the sepsis than they had realised. Over the next twenty-four hours, the team at the Freeman Hospital did everything they could to try to keep Joshua alive, but his situation became ever more desperate.

The next day, when the consultant came to see them, James knew instantly.

'He's gone,' he said, 'isn't he?'

The consultant nodded.

They went in to say goodbye to their son. The nurses had taken out all the tubes and removed the equipment. As James told me, 'He just looked like the perfect baby boy.'

A couple of years after Joshua died, my own son was born. 'There but for the grace of God,' I thought, as I listened to James tell his story. I sat with tears prickling my eyes, wondering whether this kind of thing was still happening in the health service for which I was responsible.

If James Titcombe had not been a project manager in a safety-critical industry, what happened next with the Morecambe Bay trust – indeed, the history of the modern NHS – might have turned out very differently. But because of that professional background, with his logical mind James started to make a list of all the things that had happened throughout Joshua's short life, starting with the yellow observation chart that went missing. His extraordinary battle to find out the truth lasted six years, involved the police, the courts, the senior leadership of the NHS and me as Health Secretary. James thinks he wrote over four hundred emails and letters to get to the bottom of what happened.

Mistakes are inevitable in any healthcare system. The NHS, after all, treats over one million people every thirty-six hours.[7] So what shocked me about James's story was not the existence of a mistake (even a tragic one), but the resistance to telling the truth about it to a grieving parent. To understand the lengths people will go to avoid the risk of being 'blamed' for a tragedy, it is worth looking at what James then experienced.

He started by writing a letter to Furness General Hospital. He hand-delivered it, doing everything he could to make sure it was read by the CEO. He expected all the stops to be pulled out to understand how something so catastrophic had happened. That would have been done automatically in his workplace in the nuclear industry, or indeed with many consumer complaints that were a thousand times less serious.

In fact, the opposite happened. James learned about one of the saddest ironies in modern healthcare, namely that the greater the catastrophe, the greater the temptation is to gloss over what really happened. People in hospitals are human, and they are busy. Everyone is devastated when a child dies, but that child cannot be brought back to life. So professionals often mask their discomfort about getting to the bottom of what happened by focusing their energies on patients whose lives can be saved – and sometimes allowing grieving relatives to be dismissed as unhinged or unbalanced.

James would hear reports of people saying, 'He is still coming to terms with what has happened' or 'There is nothing we can do or say that will make him better, he just needs to go through the grieving process.'

But James wasn't asking for anything more than an honest account of what happened and some reassurance that the same mistakes would not be repeated. He was met with a brick wall. The coroner refused to open an inquest, saying that Joshua had died of 'natural causes'. James pointed out to no avail that although a necrotic lung was a natural cause of death, the reason the lung became necrotic was not.

Initially, James was not even allowed to see the statements made by clinicians during the hospital's own inquiry, although he eventually forced the hospital to release them. Those statements had numerous inaccuracies. They said Joshua was pink and cried immediately when born, when in fact he was born blue and not breathing. A midwife stated that she had phoned a paediatrician for advice about Joshua, had fully informed him of Joshua's circumstances, and was told that he didn't need to be assessed – but all the paediatricians on duty that day denied such a phone call took place.[8]

He then went through the hospital's complaints process. Morecambe Bay said they would treat it as a serious incident and get clinicians from another trust to do a 'serious incident review'. But the process dragged on and the report, just seven pages, didn't emerge until three months later. It did acknowledge that Furness General had failed Joshua and that staff should have recognised Joshua's fluctuating temperature as a sign of sepsis.[9] But it didn't scratch the surface of what actually happened.

James eventually found out the full story. After exhausting the NHS complaints process, he finally persuaded the coroner to change his mind and open a full inquest. The final report was damning, accusing the midwives of collusion. James was able to prove this by uncovering a document all the midwives had used to prepare for the inquest, coaching them on the precise words and phrases to use. The coroner said it was inconceivable that eleven different midwives, all trained in different places, could claim blanket ignorance of a basic piece of knowledge, such as that a low temperature was a symptom of sepsis.

On the morning of Joshua's funeral, James went to buy some flowers. The florist asked him why, and told James her own baby had also died at Furness General. 'Just one of those things that happens,' she was told. Far from Joshua being a 'one off', as James was told, his death was the fifth incident of its kind at the hospital. Had the hospital been transparent and learned from what happened the first time, Joshua would probably be alive today.

Once it became clear there was a more systemic cover-up, James approached me as Health Secretary to ask for an independent inquiry into maternity services at the hospital. Our meeting nearly didn't happen, because, as I later learned, civil servants were reluctant for it to take place. Not because those officials weren't decent, compassionate people – but they, too, had become part of the system's defensiveness.

I agreed to meet James and to his request for an independent inquiry. I appointed Dr Bill Kirkup, an experienced obstetrician, to head it up. When his report was eventually published, it confirmed the worst fears of many families. It listed a catalogue of failings including dysfunctional management, a board completely unaware of and uninterested in what was going on, a working culture that discouraged openness, and poor oversight by the wider NHS. Up to eleven baby deaths were assessed as having been preventable.

It also became clear that a desire to sweep problems under the carpet extended well beyond the Furness General Hospital and the Morecambe Bay trust it belonged to. Professional bodies such as the Nursing and Midwifery Council (NMC) appeared to close ranks to protect the midwives involved. The Parliamentary and Health Service Ombudsman, set up to be the call of last resort, also failed to spot the issue. It was as if everyone in authority and every organisation was lined up against a father who just wanted to know why his son died.

Ultimately, therefore, it was not about rogue staff or a rogue hospital. It was about a rogue system. A rogue system that I, as Health Secretary, sat at the top of. I found James's story hard to absorb, not just because of the injustices involved, but because many of the organisations who failed him were run by people I knew well. Without exception, they were deeply committed to the NHS and its values – so why the mismatch? Why did a system set up in 1948 to embody British compassion end up – in this case – stifling a compassionate response? Why was it more natural to cover up rather than confront the many mistakes that were made?

To understand why things went wrong, we must put ourselves not just into James's shoes, but into those of the staff caring for Joshua. Not all of them were blameless – one midwife ultimately lost her licence to practise and another was suspended – but none of them wanted to be part of such a tragedy. They would have chosen their profession based on the same human instincts that motivate millions of doctors and nurses: the privilege of looking after people at their most vulnerable. That compassion comes through if you ask any doctor or nurse to recall their single most traumatic professional experience: often you end up being told heartbreaking stories of the death of a baby or child, as inevitably happens from time to time.

The trauma caused to health professionals when a patient dies is widely recognised in medicine. It is sometimes described as being a *second victim*.[10] The first victim, or set of victims, is the patient's family; but the second set is the clinical staff responsible for that patient's care. Those professionals must go home with the knowledge that if they had done things differently, their patient, perhaps a child, might still be alive. Normally they will have to go back to work the very next morning, carrying the burden of that worry on their shoulders.

One of the most powerful instincts in such situations is to seek to lessen that burden by being honest and open with families about what happened to their loved one; to learn lessons so that the same mistake is never repeated. So why would a midwife 'lose' Joshua's observation charts, which could have unlocked the biggest clues as to what went wrong?

We don't know exactly what happened, of course, and it is possible – though I believe unlikely – that the records were genuinely lost. Tampering with or destroying medical records is considered an extremely serious offence which can lead to a doctor or nurse being 'struck off'. Assuming the records were not lost, it would be easy to vilify the midwife who 'made them disappear'. Every large organisation has 'bad apples' – perhaps it was just something unacceptable that happened on this one occasion?

Unfortunately, the scale of the failures that emerged at Morecambe Bay suggests something different, namely cultural and systemic issues that went much further than any individual. And as I was to discover, those issues spread far beyond that particular hospital. I learned that modern healthcare systems, far from encouraging transparency, often – for completely unintended reasons – do the opposite. The reason is that when a mistake results in death, another emotion kicks in alongside anguish: fear.

Fear for the reputation of your unit; fear for the reputation of the hospital you work for; fear of being blamed and held responsible for a death; fear of the reaction of the victim's family; fear of lawyers and court cases; fear of losing your job; fear of being struck off the register and losing your career; and fear of multiple outside individuals or organisations who might get involved, such as – in England – the coroner, the Care Quality Commission (CQC), NHS Improvement, a Clinical Commissioning Group, the General Medical Council (GMC) or the NMC.

Those fears induce a survival instinct known as 'fight or flight'. They cause people to make unethical, but all too human, snap decisions – like hiding evidence or making false statements. And the instinct for self-preservation can also lead to subliminal changes, causing people to hide the truth from themselves with a coping mechanism called *the memory illusion*.[11]

Forensic psychologist Dr Julia Shaw describes how it works: typically, a highly stressful situation causes us to forget things that did happen or remember things that didn't. We convince ourselves that something is true or false even if the evidence suggests quite the opposite. What we end up saying is no longer even 'lying', because we actually believe it. After years of training hard to keep patients safe, frontline clinicians would not be human if they did not look for reasons why an error might not have been their fault, and start to believe them.

The memory illusion becomes even more pronounced when it is reinforced by supportive colleagues. Professor Sir Bruce Keogh was medical director of the NHS in my time and a formidable advocate of patient safety. A former cardiac surgeon, he once told me how one of his heart patients had died following a mistake he made during an operation.

'His heart was in a terrible state, Bruce, he was going to die anyway,' a colleague said to comfort him.

'Yes,' replied Bruce, 'but he wasn't going to die on Tuesday.'

As Health Secretary, dealing with such profound cultural issues in medicine felt like an impossible task. I was, however, greatly helped by the insights of the journalist and thinker Matthew Syed. In his book

Black Box Thinking, Syed shows how the airline industry faced similar issues, but none the less succeeded in massively reducing passenger fatalities – by changing a blame culture into a learning culture.[12] Despite the many differences between healthcare and aviation, it gave me hope that another industry had successfully made the journey.

Syed describes how the turning point for the airline industry was a notorious United Airlines crash in Portland, Oregon in 1978. As the plane was coming in to land, the landing wheels failed to come down. The captain, Malburn McBroom, circled the city of Portland while radioing for guidance on how to fix the landing gear. As he did so, he failed to notice the most basic thing: the fuel was running dangerously low. The plane had to crash-land. Ten people lost their lives, but because of the pilot's skill in managing a very difficult landing 179 lives were saved.

Aeronautical skill aside, running out of fuel is the one thing a pilot cannot be allowed to do. Captain McBroom ended up losing his licence and leaving the industry in disgrace. He died a broken man a few years later.

But he left a remarkable and rather surprising legacy: his shabby treatment became one of the key moments that persuaded the airline industry it needed to change its culture. If the response to near misses and accidents was always to punish the pilot, mistakes would never be learned from, only covered up.

So today, if you spot something wrong as a pilot, there are no fewer than four ways you can report it: to your airline; to your union; to your regulator; and even anonymously to a charity set up specially for the purpose. You always get a response, and unless it is gross negligence – turning up to fly a plane drunk, for example – no disciplinary process is invoked.

The result is that commercial airline fatalities have fallen globally by three quarters over a thirty-year period, even during a period when air travel increased ninefold. In 2017, the number of passenger deaths fell to zero, a remarkable achievement.[13] This has happened because the industry has been able to end its blame culture without removing accountability for passenger safety.

Not that the airline industry has resolved all its cultural issues, and fatalities rose again after 2017, largely because two Boeing 737 Max airliners crashed within five months.[14] Although eventually all Max planes were grounded in 2019, the US Congress accused Boeing of a 'culture of concealment' – which shows that even in an industry where great progress has been made there is never room for complacency.[15]

None the less, the improvement in airline passenger safety is extraordinary – and only happened when the industry changed its culture. It was American thinker David Marx who actually coined the phrase 'just culture' to describe what was needed.[16] Marx, whose background happened to be in aircraft engineering, divides human behaviour into two categories: 'normal' human behaviour, in which there is a risk of making mistakes, just because we are human; and 'reckless' behaviour, which should never be tolerated. He argues that someone who exhibits the 'normal' human tendency to make mistakes, whether a pilot, a doctor or anyone else, should be supported so that the correct lessons are learned and disseminated. But someone who behaves recklessly should be subject to a disciplinary process.

Does the lessening of sanctions for even 'normal' mistakes encourage complacency? The deterrent effect of severe punishment is the argument we generally use for giving heavy penalties to – for example – those caught using mobile phones behind the wheel of a car. It was the argument behind the disciplining of Captain McBroom. But in the case of medicine, such penalties have a particularly dangerous unintended consequence: they incentivise defensive behaviour that prevents crucial openness about what may have gone wrong. If doctors worry they could be treated like McBroom they are likely to become guarded – with the result that mistakes end up being repeated. Only a just culture prevents that happening, by properly balancing learning and accountability.

The worst culprits in the blame game, ironically, are those in my own profession: politicians. Week after week as Health Secretary, I found myself blaming and being blamed – in equal measure – by Andy Burnham, the Shadow Health Secretary. Andy knew his stuff, having been Health Secretary under the previous Labour government, but I faced a constant deluge of bogus attacks in the Commons about a 'toxic mix of cuts and privatisation'.[17] Neither charge was true, but because of the ferocity of the attacks I fought fire with fire by holding Andy himself to account for his failure to tackle what happened at Mid Staffs. The result was a big escalation in the rivalry between us, which at one point even led to him initiating legal action against me for tweeting about a *Daily Mail* headline.[18]

We were both sucked into our own version of the blame game – something that can hardly have inspired doctors and nurses trying to foster a more positive culture in the NHS. I discovered for myself – just like many doctors, nurses and midwives – that when you are under attack a survival instinct kicks in and you fight back. But if that leads to unedifying spats in the political arena, in medicine it creates an additional problem: making it impossible to learn from mistakes in a way that stops tragedies being repeated. So how do you dismantle the blame culture in modern medicine?

We need to remove the threat of being fired or found guilty of clinical negligence from doctors, nurses and midwives who make the kind of errors that any human being could make. There should be no lessening of accountability for reckless behaviour or gross negligence, but a proper differentiation in law between such behaviour and ordinary human error, as happens in sectors like the airline industry. By doing this we would not just be treating frontline staff more fairly, but also be creating space for people to learn from mistakes. Rather than penalising openness – as we do now – we should reward it. The principal penalties should exist for people who do the opposite, sweeping mistakes under the carpet, preventing lessons from being learned and causing tragedies to be repeated.

I took a step towards this by introducing something called a 'duty of candour',[19] which requires hospitals to be open with families if mistakes have been made. It has helped in certain situations, but in the end, there is little hospital managers can do if their own staff do not feel able to be open about potentially fatal errors. And for ordinary doctors and nurses, the price of speaking out can still feel higher than the transparency necessary to improve systems. Added to which, the laws around clinical negligence are applied inconsistently around the country. If clinicians cannot be wholly sure where the line will be drawn, they are unlikely to feel able to speak openly. Hence the need for professional codes of conduct and, if necessary, legislation to resolve these issues and make it safer to speak out.

Even without such improvements, there are a few encouraging signs that the blame culture in modern medicine is beginning to change. And in the end there was one positive thing to come out of Joshua Titcombe's sad story. Morecambe Bay was put into 'special measures' under the new hospital inspection regime introduced after Mid Staffs.[20] The recently appointed chief executive, Jackie Daniel, was a former nurse with a strong interest in improving clinical standards. She set about a root-and-branch transformation of the safety culture in the hospital. It was, she told me, 'the most complete rebuild of any job I've had to do.'

Listening to her describe what she had to do gives important clues as to what had gone wrong. The management team she inherited was focused not on issues relating to patient care, but on organisational goals. These included becoming what is called a 'Foundation Trust' (which gives hospitals more autonomy) and with it the right to take over the running of other hospitals. Jackie put in place new leadership and set up partnerships with hospitals in Manchester, Salford and Preston that had a better track record in the quality of their patient care.

She focused on changing the hospital's blame culture into an improvement ethos, with staff closely involved in her reforms. She also engaged with families who had suffered, refusing to treat them as 'troublesome' and recognising the anguish and suffering they had experienced. She charged an inspiring new head of midwifery, Sascha Wells, to turn around the troubled maternity services.

Jackie invested heavily in mechanisms to make it easier for staff to speak out about any concerns. They were trained in a no-blame approach to improving processes known as 'human factors thinking'. Nurses were encouraged to spend time at the end of a shift reflecting on ways to improve the care they had given in a structured 'mop-up' session known as a 'Schwartz round'. Mediators were used to bring staff and families affected by the maternity tragedies together, and a board committee met in public to go through the lessons that had been learned.

The results were transformational – and came more quickly than many predicted. From the seriously dysfunctional and dangerous maternity unit described in the Kirkup Report, in 2016 maternity services across Morecambe Bay were rated as 'good',[21] indeed considered some of the best in the NHS. Their performance in the annual NHS staff survey went from the bottom quartile to the top.[22] Although the trust has had more problems recently,[23] the transformation showed

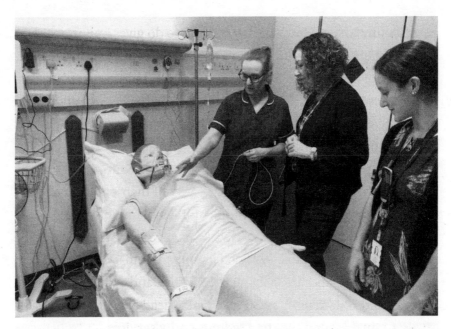

Dame Jackie Daniel on the rounds

how quickly it is possible to change a blame culture into something more positive.

Thanks to James Titcombe's campaigning, I agreed to set up an independent organisation to perform no-fault investigations into unexpected deaths in the NHS. It was modelled on the approach taken by the airline industry, where an organisation called the Air Accidents Investigation Branch (the AAIB) can undertake immediate and thorough investigations. The identities of any witnesses are protected, so they feel able to speak freely. The new organisation for the NHS is called the Healthcare Safety Investigation Branch.[24] It is in the process of being put on a statutory footing so that people who give evidence to its investigations have legal protection.

The NHS has also set up a system to make it easier for frontline staff to speak out if they have concerns about patient safety. Because people are sometimes reluctant to talk to their line manager (not least because their line manager may be the subject of those concerns), every hospital now has an independent person whom staff can approach confidentially, known as a Freedom to Speak Up Guardian.[25] That 'guardian' has direct access to the hospital chief executive to communicate any concerns – and there are more than three hundred such Guardians across the NHS. Under Jackie Daniel's leadership, Morecambe Bay was one of the first trusts in the NHS to set up such a system.

But perhaps the most remarkable outcome was something much more personal.

A midwife involved in Joshua Titcombe's care was heavily criticised by the NMC, which concluded that her mistakes were serious enough to warrant a temporary suspension.[26] That meant she could not practise – and the hospital had to decide whether to dismiss her. But before making their final decision, they did something very unusual: they asked James if he would be willing to meet her.

It gave James a real dilemma. In all his years of campaigning, the only time he had been in a room with the staff involved with Joshua's care was at his inquest and at formal 'fitness to practise' hearings. These were cold and clinical legal settings, and this would be something very different. None the less, James agreed to the meeting.

He worked out carefully what he wanted to say, namely, that while he didn't blame the midwife personally for the mistakes made in Joshua's care, the lack of honesty about what happened afterwards had a huge impact on him and his family – and had made him incredibly angry that Joshua's life seemed to matter so little.

When he walked into the room and sat with the midwife, he got through half of what he wanted to say... but couldn't get any further. The midwife broke down in tears and said that she had blamed herself for what happened every single day since Joshua had died. She said she wished she had done things differently, and would carry on doing so for the rest of her life. It was not fake or rehearsed – and James's image of her as an uncaring person melted away. They cried together and had a hug.

Following the meeting, the hospital decided not to dismiss the midwife, and she was able to go back to practising at the end of her temporary suspension. That surely was the right outcome – both for her and for James. But why had it taken so long to get there and at such great cost?

As James now says, 'The most important legacy of Joshua's tragedy is that the trust that caused his death improved, although recent developments show there is no room for complacency. Whilst we can't bring Joshua back, I am confident that the circumstances that led to his death could not happen today.'

Unfortunately, as I was to discover, a lot more needs to be done to make that true. And when it comes to the NHS, tackling staff shortages is right at the top of the list.

2

Short-Staffing

I arrived at the Department of Health for a typically busy day. I was focused on drafting announcements about access to the NHS for migrants, preparing to be questioned in the House of Commons and mulling over follow-up actions from a Cabinet presentation. But all these issues were shunted to the back of my mind when I read my daily letter. It came from someone called Eve Sambrook.

Eve was an ordinary person who had lived an extraordinary life. Her father was a young Chinese aristocrat who came to London in the 1920s, fell in love with a chambermaid and took her back to China, where Eve was born. His family disapproved of the match so Eve returned to London with her mother. Then, as a young adult, she smuggled herself to China to join the Communist Revolution in 1949. She became a major in the Red Army, where her job was to broadcast Mao's propaganda on Radio Peking. She fell out of favour with her Communist masters, however, and returned to the UK just as the Cultural Revolution was gathering steam.

Back in the UK, she met her husband John – a fellow left-wing radical who had escaped from Nazi Germany and wrote for the *Daily Worker*. He was the love of her life, and although they were both firebrand journalists she ended up in a rather more traditional role, as headmistress of a village school in the West Country. After retiring they moved to London to be near their children. Then, at the age of eighty-four, John became ill with liver damage and was admitted to a respected London hospital. They received the bad news that he had disappearing liver ducts, for which there is no cure.

Life or death in that London hospital ward seemed to be a matter of chance. A piece of plastic that said 'nil by mouth', meaning patients had to be fed intravenously, had been kicked around on the floor of the ward for two days. Eve kept picking it up and putting it by the bin for one of the nurses to take away. Once, when Eve went out to make a cup of tea, she came back to find that an agency nurse had pinned the notice above John's bed. John needed a high-protein diet to survive, so it was a potentially catastrophic mistake. Thankfully, Eve spotted it.

Other simple procedures were neglected. John was put on a nasal feed during the night, but he could eat smaller quantities normally during the day. But the timings were never observed. Different agency nurses came during the day and at all hours, wreaking havoc with John's diet. When the feed was empty, Eve had to beg someone to change it. In the end, she did it herself.

Some of John's medicines were supposed to be given before he ate, others two hours afterwards, when he had digested his meal. But often all the medicines were dished out together, with no care given as to what should be taken when.

The next part of the story I remember Eve telling me herself. It was so shocking that I had invited her to my office to tell me again in person. She recounted that one evening, as she was at the hospital tending to John, she needed a shower and change of clothes. So she permitted herself a short break from John's bedside and went to a nearby chain hotel to freshen up.

She came back at 4 a.m. to check that John was okay.

She found him lying naked on a rubber mat on the floor. He was soaked in urine and faeces, with his clothes spread out around him. He was shaking with cold, in a foetal position, with a cold blast of air coming from the air conditioning right down on top of him. Forcing herself to focus, she rushed to his side. Her voice rising with panic, she asked a passing nurse for a change of sheets.

The nurse refused.

'We don't change sheets till ten o'clock in the morning,' she said, in a matter-of-fact way. It would be even longer before they changed the blankets, as that only happened twice a week.

In despair, Eve wrapped John up in her pashmina to try to keep him warm. Then she started doing what she could to clean him up, but it was too late. John never recovered. Eve took a chair beside his bed and slept on it, fearful of leaving his side again even for a few minutes.

When he was eventually discharged, Eve knew he was really being sent home to die. But even then, the system proved a battle. He was discharged at 1 p.m. but didn't arrive home until nearly 10 p.m., not in an ambulance but in an unheated van. Five days after his eighty-fifth birthday, John Sambrook died.

I was the Health Secretary when it happened, so John died on my watch. Despite that, Eve was generous with me personally when I met her. But none the less, my head was spinning trying to understand how this could possibly happen – not at Mid Staffs, where I knew there were big management problems, but at a respected London hospital. Was it an uncaring nurse? Management oversight? Or a lack of staff and resources? As Health Secretary, I needed to know the answer.

I was conscious that I had only heard one side of the story when I read Eve's letter, so I asked the chief executive of the hospital to come in at the same time as Eve. He was experienced, and the hospital was considered well run. In the meeting he apologised to Eve, and seemed genuinely contrite. I had many subsequent dealings with that CEO, and came to believe he was indeed an excellent leader. I also have no doubt that the hospital did everything possible after that meeting to make sure John's story was not repeated.

But why, when Eve had found John covered in faeces, had she been told nothing could be done? Why were new sheets not available for five hours? Why would anyone in a caring profession refuse such a basic human request? There was an awkward silence around the table in my office when I asked these questions. The CEO's face looked blank. He then sheepishly admitted they had not spoken to the individual, because she was an agency nurse.

It troubled me that they had not bothered to track her down, even though they knew they were meeting the Health Secretary. I began to worry that it may not have been such an unusual occurrence. Then I asked myself what that nurse would have said if someone *had* tracked her down.

I'll never know for sure what her answer would have been, but I suspect a different story would have emerged. She might have described a night shift where she was run ragged looking after different patients. She might have been on her own or with minimal additional support. She might, perhaps, have been rushing to an emergency when she was stopped by Eve asking for clean sheets. There may not have been any clean sheets available anyway. Rather than her being hard-hearted, it is more likely that the situation she had to cope with led to the behaviour she exhibited. Better staffing levels might not have prevented or solved the problem, but would at least have given her more time to address it.

———

As we saw in the first chapter, a blame culture stops people learning from things that go wrong. But if there are nationwide staff shortages, such things are more likely to happen. In this chapter we look at why safe levels of staffing matter – and some of the pitfalls when you try to make it happen.

It takes three years to train a nurse, seven years to train a doctor and eleven years to train a consultant. Any plan to increase staffing levels takes a long time – far longer than the horizons of many stressed politicians.

You can of course import clinical staff – indeed our failure over decades to train enough doctors and nurses is one of the reasons why in 2019 28% of NHS doctors and 18% of NHS nurses were non-British nationals.[1] They are generally brilliant recruits who plug a vital gap, and often come from developing countries. But how can we justify recruiting 302 NHS staff from Somalia when they are desperately needed at home?[2]

The NHS should keep its doors open for the brightest and best from all over the world, but the get-out-of-jail-free card of international recruitment – upon which the NHS has always depended – is running dry. Developing countries are busy expanding their own healthcare systems, and everyone has a post-Covid pandemic backlog. The result is a global shortage of professionals – and this will reach around 18 million by 2030, according to the WHO.[3] Any large healthcare system therefore has no choice but to train up its own clinicians.

But predicting how many doctors and nurses you will need in a decade's time is notoriously difficult. Innovations in treatment and medicine constantly change staffing requirements. Scandals like Mid Staffs create unexpected surges in demand for staff. Whole new areas open up with specific staffing requirements, such as cognitive behaviour therapy in mental health. On the other hand, the need to provide care for an ageing population has been no secret to anyone – and you would have expected policymakers to recommend a long-term, sustained increase in the NHS workforce to address it. In fact, when I became Health Secretary in 2012, not only was there no such plan, we were going in the opposite direction. Nurse numbers were down, doctor training places were being cut, and the plan – believe it or not – was to keep on *reducing* staff levels.

This was down to a combination of NHS orthodoxy, professional lobbying and government expediency. The orthodoxy was that health-care systems around the world would need less staff because of shorter hospital stays, and more 'day cases' as opposed to overnight admissions. Big improvements in surgery now make it possible to do procedures such as biopsies, endoscopies and keyhole surgery in a single day without needing a patient to stay overnight. That has meant that the average length of hospital stays in the UK has reduced from 8.4 to 4.5 days over the last two decades[4] – a positive change, but one also used to justify significant staffing reductions. Principally for that reason, as recently as a decade ago NHS trusts believed they would need about 5,000 *fewer* nurses in the following five years. None, of course, would say that now.

The professional lobbying came from a long-established view that it was essential to be able to guarantee every doctor a job at the end of their training. Organisations like the BMA resisted the expansion of medical school training places for many years, arguing strongly against 'the overproduction of doctors with limited career opportunities.'[5]

Nor did governments object, given the constant pressure for efficiency savings following the financial crisis of 2008. In such a climate, big rises in staff numbers were not on the table. But the Francis Report into the Mid Staffs scandal made it clear that staffing shortfalls were a serious issue.[6] I looked carefully at introducing mandatory staffing ratios on wards, a solution championed powerfully by campaigners like Julie Bailey, who lost her mother at Mid Staffs.[7] But that approach was strongly opposed by many hospital chief nurses, who felt that arbitrary legal ratios would limit their flexibility to move staff around a hospital to where they were most needed. It is also not clear where the extra nurses would come from.

I didn't realise it at the time, but that debate reflected one of the key dilemmas in patient safety: why, some ask, can hospitals not be run like airlines? When an airline doesn't have enough staff to fly safely, the aircraft does not take off. Should it not be the same for hospitals? The two industries cannot, of course, be treated identically. No one dies if a plane fails to take off – but if a short-staffed A & E closes its doors, the next patient to arrive is put in danger. Even with inadequate numbers of staff, surgeries and hospitals still have to operate – with the price paid by exhausted doctors and patients whose care is less than fully safe. But even if mandating safe staffing levels airline-style is not practical in the short term, and may never be feasible for walk-in emergency care, the rigorous principles that underlie it have merit as a longer-term objective.

In my response to the Francis Inquiry, I did not have the luxury of time – I needed to act right away. So I did something quite straightforward. I simply asked – required – every hospital to publish, monthly, the number of nurses they employed on each of their wards.[8]

The line marked with circles in Fig. 1 represents the number of nurses employed to care for adults in the first two years that Cameron was Prime Minister. The numbers show a gentle decline, because of that prevailing orthodoxy about reducing the requirement for staff thanks to advances in surgery (and no doubt the pressure to produce efficiency savings). This is also reflected in the grey line with diamonds, which shows the projections of future nurse numbers NHS hospitals

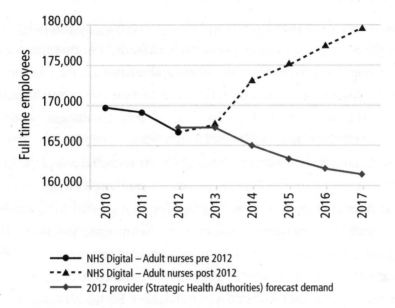

Fig. 1: Actual nurse numbers vs projected nurse numbers 2011 to 2017

thought they would need going forward. Then, in 2013, ward-by-ward transparency was introduced. The dashed line with triangles shows what *actually* happened to nurse numbers: a significant increase. As a result, the number of ward nurses went up by around 13,500 over the following five years. Perhaps unsurprisingly, patient satisfaction with hospital care also rose to record levels.

This didn't happen because of instructions or targets. It happened simply because people were asked to publish the number of nurses they were using – the soft power of transparency. So wards such as the one John Sambrook was treated in saw an increase in nursing staff – as, in fact, did wards in every hospital in the country. But all health secretaries end up getting their fingers burned with the unintended consequences of their decisions, and I was no exception.

First, the positive: the overall number of frontline clinicians increased by around 45,000, including 11,000 more nurses,[9] because of the transparency measures introduced. They included not just publication of ward staffing numbers but also a new, independent inspection regime focused on the safety and quality of care. But then came the unintended consequences: because hospitals wanted even more than 11,000 more nurses, they pulled in staff from community nursing, district nursing and mental health settings. Those community settings then saw their nurse numbers fall: I had squeezed the balloon in one place only to see a bubble emerge somewhere else.

The impact of poor workforce planning is not just felt in wards and surgeries – it also hits healthcare organisations hard, by inflating the salaries and rates paid to locum doctors and agency nurses who end up filling the gaps. The NHS spends an extraordinary £6 billion every year on temporary staff[10] – an outrageous waste of money that amounts to more than the entire budget of several smaller government departments. Such staff are quasi-permanent, but the higher rates they command as 'temporary' are both expensive and divisive: why should one nurse be paid twice as much as another when they have the same experience and are working the very same shift?

The NHS is conditioned to ask ministers for money every time a request is made to improve services. But extra money has little impact if there aren't enough staff to deliver that improvement. There is no point giving an extra billion pounds to cut waiting lists or improve care, if you don't have a billion pounds' worth of additional doctors and nurses to spend it on – and if you don't, the extra money will simply inflate the salaries of the existing workforce, particularly agency staff and locums.

Some have tried to get around this issue by contracting the private sector to do additional work for the NHS. Unfortunately this doesn't work either, because independent hospitals fish from the same pool of doctors for their workforce – indeed, they employ NHS doctors for much of their work. Over-reliance on the private sector therefore sucks doctors and nurses out of NHS hospitals, making waiting lists even longer. The only answer is to consider properly the entire capacity of the system, whether NHS or independent. Because we have failed to do that kind of capacity planning, we continue to have lower numbers of doctors per head than many comparable countries, as the graph below shows.

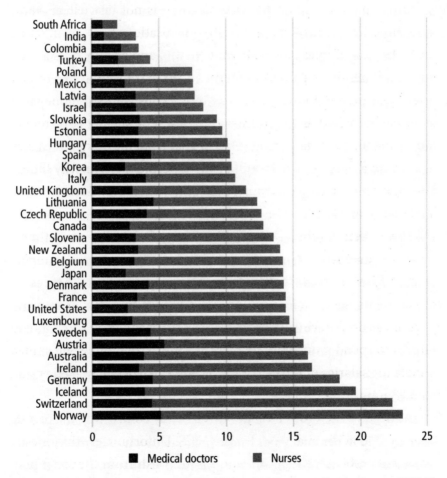

Fig. 2: Doctors and nurses per 1,000 inhabitants, 2020 or latest figures (Source: OECD[11])

This relatively low number of doctors makes daily work extremely pressured. Frontline staff are increasingly experiencing what is called 'burnout', characterised by the WHO as 'feelings of energy depletion or exhaustion', 'increased mental distance from one's job, or feelings of negativism or cynicism related to one's job' and 'reduced professional efficacy'.[12] In the latest NHS staff survey, around 40% of frontline staff say they have been unable to function properly at work because of stress.[13] As a result, many then choose to reduce their hours and work part-time, but in doing so – for perfectly understandable reasons – they exacerbate the pressure on their colleagues even more.

Addressing such issues is fraught with difficulty. In 2015, I publicly promised to recruit 5,000 more GPs by 2020.[14] I was aware of the pressures in general practice and assured by officials in my department that we could meet this important pledge. I wanted to deliver it not just to reduce that pressure, but also to allow a return to a more personalised service, where patients could go back to having their 'own GP' – something I believed was both appealing to patients and clinically safer. However, I failed badly in that pledge: by the time I left the role in 2018 there were just under 300 more GPs.[15]

The reason for that failure is instructive: I had pulled a lever I could control, namely the number of medical students we trained who went into general practice. Their numbers rose to record levels – more than 3,000 a year.[16] But while the number of new GPs was increasing, the number choosing to work part-time or retire early also increased by about the same number. The result was that after a lot of effort we were back to square one.

However, a decision I took in 2016 had more success. I persuaded Theresa May, in her first major health policy decision as Prime Minister, to increase the number of doctors we trained by a quarter.[17] It was a decision that led to the opening of five new medical schools, but would only reap dividends many years hence (when, as it turned out, neither of us would be in office). To her credit, May made the decision enthusiastically, because as Home Secretary she had despaired at the number of visas she was having to offer medics from overseas given the number of people wanting to become doctors in the UK. The following year, she went even further and agreed to do the same for the number of trainee nurses and midwives.[18]

So if there was one thing I wish I had known at the start of my time as Health Secretary, it is the importance of long-term workforce planning. Too often, the number of doctors and nurses we train is the very last thing discussed in spending review discussions between a Chancellor and a Health Secretary. Given that any decision taken will not impact the NHS for around eight years, it is rarely a priority for either. Even worse, because it does not count as 'frontline' NHS spending, it is not ring-fenced in the core NHS budget but contained in a budget held separately by the Department of Health, which is politically much easier to cut.

Even now, when we face a huge backlog of operations after the pandemic, it is not clear that these lessons have been learned. The government has introduced an 'NHS visa' – but as we have seen, the immigration tap is now running dry. It also voted down an amendment to the 2022 Health and Care Bill that would have seen regular, independent forecasts published of the number of doctors and nurses we should be training.[19] At the time of writing there are 99,000 vacancies,[20] with the Royal Colleges saying we need 500 more obstetricians, 1,400 more anaesthetists, 1,900 more radiologists, 2,000 more midwives, up to 2,500 more A & E consultants, 2,500 more GPs and 39,000 more nurses.[21] The government has promised a long-term workforce plan, but because it won't be independent it will simply trumpet the numbers they decide to train. It will not answer the crucial question as to whether those numbers are enough – and even more disappointingly, it will be published after the big spending decisions have been taken.

The solution is to ask an independent body to monitor and publish the long-term workforce requirements of both the health and social care systems. It should give a balanced verdict on the number of doctors, nurses, allied health professionals and care workers needed in every specialty over the next five, ten and twenty years, with those numbers updated at least every two years to account for changes in either demand or technology. It should also give a fair judgement as to whether we are training enough people to deliver those numbers. In other words, it should keep the system honest – just as the independent Office for Budget Responsibility (OBR) does for the Treasury in budgets. Since the OBR was set up, we have ended the regular claims that Treasury ministers were altering forecasts or 'cooking the books' for party political purposes. We need the same rigour with respect to ministerial pledges that we have 'enough' doctors and nurses. Ultimately, such reforms are the only way to make stories like that of John Sambrook less likely.

The last time I saw Eve Sambrook, she told me her sister had just died from lung cancer. She had endured a painful life, crippled with rheumatoid arthritis, but her NHS care was exemplary in every respect. On the way out, she paused, the former Red Army major composing herself. 'I just wish it had been the same for John,' she said.

3

Money

During my time in office, I was responsible for a pot of money called the Cancer Drugs Fund.[1] It was set up by the then Prime Minister, David Cameron, to speed up patients' access to the latest cancer drugs – a big issue in the run-up to the 2010 election. But the fund became a victim of its own success and started going massively over budget. Initially, we increased the budget from £200 million to £280 million, and then even further, to £340 million.[2] Eventually we started having to divert money from other vital areas of frontline healthcare to fund it.

My officials made a sensible – if sensitive – proposal to delist several of the less effective drugs, meaning that they would no longer be eligible for support from the fund. None of the drugs were cures, and they generally only extended life for a few extra months. Given the pressure the overspend was putting on other budgets, I accepted the proposal.

A few months later, a young couple came to see me in my constituency surgery. The husband had bowel cancer. My face fell as he told me that the drug he needed to keep him alive for a short while was no longer available on the NHS. It was one of the drugs I had delisted.

'I just want to be alive to see my daughter take her GCSEs,' he told me.

I looked them both in the eye and told them exactly what had happened, including the fact that I personally had made the decision to delist the drug. They could not have been more generous and understanding. In the end, I found a way for that father to get hold of the drug he needed – but the encounter remained with me. I had been confronted with the consequences of one of my own decisions – forced on me by a need to save money.

Any examination of how to prevent avoidable harm and death in a modern healthcare system needs to consider the issue of resources. We have looked at the way blame gets in the way of learning and how staffing shortfalls can cause unsafe care. But staff cost money – typically around two thirds of the total budget of a healthcare organisation. So is safe care something you just have to buy?

In this chapter, we look in more detail at the importance of and cost associated with adequate resourcing. We discover two things, one obvious, the other more surprising. The obvious point is that if staff levels are not safe it costs money to recruit more. The surprise is that, having done so, healthcare organisations that focus on providing safe care find that it is much, much cheaper to deliver.

That applies at an organisational level – say to a hospital or a GP surgery. But in the case of the UK the money such organisations receive is largely determined by how much funding is going into the NHS at a national level. And here there is another fact that may surprise some readers: the NHS is not actually underfunded when compared to the proportion of GDP allocated to healthcare systems in similar countries. We sit at around the average for Western European countries and for the broader group of developed countries that belong to the OECD.

Country	Total healthcare expenditure as % of GDP	Government spending and compulsory health insurance as % of GDP	Voluntary spending (voluntary health insurance and private funds such as households' out-of-pocket payments, NGOs and private corporations) as % of GDP
France	11.1%	9.3%	1.8%
Germany	12.5%	10.7%	1.9%
Italy	9.7%	7.4%	2.3%
Japan	11.0%	9.3%	1.8%
UK	12.8%	10.4%	2.3%
US	16.8%	13.9%	2.9%

Table 1: 2019/20 health spending as a percentage of GDP, broken down into total spending, government/compulsory spending and voluntary spending (Source: OECD[3])

There is, however, an important caveat to those numbers, particularly when it comes to the prevention of avoidable harm and death. Spending a broadly similar proportion of your national income as other countries does not necessarily mean you are spending enough. Indeed, absolute spending per head remains significantly lower than in countries that we often compare ourselves to directly, such as Germany (22% lower) or France (5% lower). Those absolute differences of course make a big difference when it comes to funding state-of-the-art cancer machines or additional doctors. So how much is 'enough'? To answer that you need to know about the quality of care that is delivered and the efficiency with which resources are spent.

Unfortunately, these are extremely difficult things to compare between countries. When it comes to outcomes in cancer, for example, the NHS lags behind countries like Denmark and Australia. But when it comes to the ability of poorer people to access good-quality care, surely a central objective for any civilised country, the NHS scores better than anywhere else. Only one organisation has tried to make such comparisons in a balanced way over many years, the New York-based

Commonwealth Fund. As you can see from Table 2, it gives the NHS a relatively high overall ranking – fourth out of eleven countries, behind Norway, the Netherlands and Australia but ahead of both France and Germany. The NHS scores particularly well for the equity of its system, its low administration costs and the speed and safety of care. But it does poorly when it comes to healthcare outcomes and the number of early deaths that could have been avoided by a health system intervention. That may be linked to high differences in disease-free life expectancy between wealthier and poorer parts of the country. Such issues are extremely important to address but not necessarily within the ability of the NHS to deal with on its own.

I concluded early on that the NHS needed more funding after seeing the poor care caused by short-staffing in Mid Staffs and other hospitals. But what allowed me to win the argument inside government was something totally different: the demographic and scientific changes that are causing every country looked at by the Commonwealth Fund to increase its health spending.

	NOR	NETH	AUS	UK	GER	NZ	SWE	FRA	SWIZ	CAN	US
Overall ranking	1	2	3	4	5	6	7	8	9	10	11
Access to care	2	1	8	4	3	5	6	7	10	9	11
Care process	8	3	6	5	9	1	11	10	7	4	2
Administrative efficiency	1	8	2	4	9	3	5	6	10	7	11
Equity	8	5	1	4	2	9	6	7	3	10	11
Health care outcomes	2	4	1	9	7	8	5	6	3	10	11

Table 2: Commonwealth Fund international ranking of healthcare systems (Source: Commonwealth Fund[4])

Such changes are so stark that they are difficult for even the most hardened of Treasury ministers to dismiss. Until the Covid-19 pandemic, life expectancy in the UK was going up by about one year for every eight that we live.[5] That is good news for most of us but very bad news for anyone trying to control healthcare spend. That's because those additional years of life are not necessarily healthy, meaning that healthcare systems have to cope with many more people with long-term conditions such as dementia, diabetes and arthritis. Currently around 10% of the UK population has four or more such conditions, a number that is forecast to nearly double within two decades.[6] Looking after people with such conditions is expensive – even now, long-term conditions account for half of all GP appointments and around 70% of hospital bed days.[7]

Those increases in life expectancy are being fuelled by the progress of science – where the pace of change is quickening. One example is dementia: when I was Health Secretary, David Cameron and Barack Obama launched a challenge to find a cure for that horrible disease by 2025.[8] We may just get there, which would be wonderful for those with the condition – but not so wonderful for the NHS drugs bill, which will also be having to fund other scientific breakthroughs and new priorities such as the vaccine research and production we will need after Covid-19.

You might imagine, given that health and social care represents more than 40% of day-to-day government spending,[9] that there would be a rigorous, logical process to get to the bottom of such issues and calculate the exact amount needed. But I found the opposite to be the case – indeed the process through which a health secretary secures extra funding is surprisingly haphazard. Because of its central importance to safe care for patients, let's take a moment to look at how that happens in the UK.

The starting point is that the Department of Health is always viewed by the Treasury as the most troublesome government department: others would haggle for months over £10 or £20 million – but for the NHS you would need to add not one but two or three noughts to those numbers. A small change in health spending, by far the largest single item if you exclude the benefits bill, has a major impact on the national accounts. Even worse, from the Treasury's point of view, is that like Oliver Twist we always came back for more. Timing was everything, if you were to be successful in overcoming those deep suspicions – and there is no better moment than just before a general election.

In the run-up to the 2015 election, Simon Stevens, the then NHS England chief executive, cleverly laid the ground for a funding increase by publishing a plan for the NHS called the Five Year Forward View.[10] His plan was widely welcomed, but he also let it be known quietly that it had a delivery cost of at least £8 billion of extra funding a year. Simon was a formidable operator with a profound commitment to the NHS. By putting a price tag on his plans, however uncomfortable it was for the government, he took them a step closer to fruition.

Six months on we were in the midst of the election campaign, and the Conservatives were being hammered by Labour leader Ed Miliband on NHS funding. I sensed the opportunity, so went to meet the Chancellor, George Osborne, in his office at No. 11 Downing Street. It was a meeting I will never forget. I was ushered into his office, where, far from giving me his full attention, he was in the middle of a haircut. In fairness, he was fitting me into a packed campaign day, but conversations with colleagues were being carried on with the same insouciance that Churchill presumably displayed when giving instructions from his bed in his pyjamas. Because it was an election campaign meeting, there were no Treasury officials present – something that turned out to be of great significance.

My pitch to George, as the scissors snipped away, was political: Labour had not signed up to Simon Stevens's £8 billion request. If we signed up to it we could kill off Ed Miliband's attack and turn a weakness into a strength. George, perhaps the smartest political operator I ever met, bought the idea. It was announced a couple of days later. Unfortunately for the country's coffers (but not the NHS), in the heat of the moment it appeared to be overlooked that the NHS had already got £2 billion of the £8 billion in the Autumn Statement six months earlier. So when the government promised 'an additional £8 billion' we secured £2 billion more for the NHS – just like that. That famous comment attributed to Senator Everett Dirksen rang in my ears: 'A billion here, a billion there, soon we'll be talking real money.'

The second opportunity I had to pitch for more funding came three years later, by which time Theresa May was Prime Minister. Again, Simon Stevens played a crucial role in laying the ground. Ahead of the budget in December 2017, he made an audacious public demand for an extra £4 billion.[11] It was in government eyes also an outrageous thing to do – not because the money wasn't needed, but because he broke the convention that public servants should do their lobbying in private. He also did so just a few weeks ahead of the Budget, when he must have known the spending envelope would already have been decided. None the less, the row his intervention caused started a crucial debate inside Whitehall about NHS funding.

Once again, timing was critical. There was no election this time, but six months later would see the seventieth anniversary of the founding of the NHS. All of us in government knew there would be a huge national focus on our most loved national institution – something greatly to the advantage of a Health Secretary seeking more funding. I sent letter after letter to the Prime Minister arguing for more money, stressing both the intrinsic need and the presentational risks of not doing so. I argued that we should settle the issue once and for all with a ten-year plan backed up by a long-term funding settlement. I had strong support from the then Cabinet Secretary, Jeremy Heywood – made all the more poignant because he was fighting a losing battle against cancer at the time.

In the many discussions we had, there was one moment in particular when I knew I had won. In a conversation between May and the Chancellor, Philip Hammond, the Prime Minister suddenly said, 'Let's face it, Philip, the NHS *does* need more money!' To her credit, she had grasped the issue. Cabinet ministers – including chancellors – read such signs from their boss very clearly.

A deal was finally thrashed out at a meeting in her office, although without her being present. Alongside me were Simon Stevens, Philip Hammond and the top Treasury officials. Two or three times during that long afternoon, it looked like the talks would collapse – on one occasion I had to coax Simon back to the table; on another, Philip. But in the end, the NHS got an agreement for a 3.4% annual real-term increase over each of the following five years.[12] It was less than the annual percentage increases a decade earlier, but as a five-year commitment still the largest single increase in NHS history, equivalent to around 1% of Britain's GDP.

Whether it was enough I will leave to others to judge – and in the case of social care, which I was unable to settle at the same time, there clearly remains unfinished business. But what surely everyone can agree is that the process by which the biggest single budget in government is settled is far too random – decided on the back of headlines, elections and anniversaries rather than on the basis of rational calculations of demand and cost. The costs of a pandemic may not be predictable, but those associated with an ageing society most certainly are. Many of those expenditures, such as training enough staff, building new hospitals and investing in new IT systems, need to be planned well outside a five-year parliamentary cycle. Surely we need to find a longer-term, more strategic approach to funding our health and social care systems.

Let me return to the central question as to whether safe care that prioritises the reduction of avoidable harm and death is ultimately more expensive. It is of course true that organisations with unsafe staffing levels have to spend more on bringing their staff numbers up to appropriate levels. But ironically the opposite then becomes true: when appropriate levels of staffing are in place, safer care becomes vastly cheaper to deliver. Let me explain why – and how, because of the way it is regulated and funded, the NHS is perhaps the only organisation in the world that can prove this beyond doubt.

There are two things that are very unusual in the way the English NHS is organised, compared to other healthcare systems. Firstly, hospitals are paid standardised prices (known as the national tariff) for their services. That means that across the whole country the same rate is paid by the NHS, for example, for a hip replacement or an A & E attendance. Secondly, every hospital is inspected independently for the safety of its care by the CQC. It therefore becomes possible to compare the quality of care between organisations that are paid broadly the same amount for the same work. You can also compare the financial health of hospitals delivering safer care with those delivering less safe care.

The graph in Fig. 3 compares the finances of hospitals ranked 'good' or 'outstanding' for the quality of their care with those ranked as 'requiring improvement' or 'inadequate', after the first round of independent quality inspections was completed in 2015.[13]

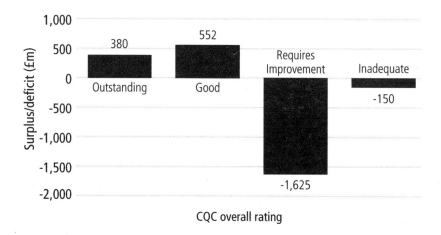

Fig. 3: Surplus/deficit of hospitals for each overall CQC rating

A very clear pattern emerges. On average, the better hospitals have a financial surplus and the poorer ones have a deficit (these figures are from before the Covid-19 pandemic, and so characteristic of more normal times). Almost without exception, hospitals delivering the best care also have the best finances. How can that be, given that all hospitals are paid standardised tariffs?

The answer is something every doctor or nurse intuitively understands, namely that poor care is about the most expensive care you can give. If someone acquires an infection during their hospital stay, or has a fall that could have been avoided, they end up staying in hospital for longer. That costs both the hospital and the NHS more.

The annual cost to the NHS caused by older people having falls, whether at home or in hospital, has been estimated at a hefty £2 billion a year.[14] Another NHS body has calculated that the average additional cost of a fall while in NHS care is £2,600 per incident – caused by longer hospital stays, additional surgery, or treatment and litigation costs.[15] Around a quarter of that cost is borne directly by the hospital.

Another example is infections such as MRSA or C. difficile (C. diff).

Every year around 300,000 patients acquire such an infection during a hospital stay in England, something the National Institute for Health and Care Excellence (NICE) estimates costs the NHS a staggering £1 billion per annum.[16] By definition, hospitals with higher levels of infection bear higher levels of cost. Likewise when a patient is given the wrong drug, something which can be fatal. Adverse drug reactions cost the NHS nearly £100 million a year, according to a study run by the universities of York, Sheffield and Manchester, something that would be of little surprise to frontline clinicians.[17]

Halving the incidence of hospital-acquired infections would fund 5,000 more consultants or 15,000 more nurses across the NHS.[18] In effect, that is exactly what happens at the better hospitals. Because they spend less time and money on dealing with the consequences of poor care, they are able to invest more of both in delivering better care. Conversely, the hospitals where adverse events happen more frequently end up with less money to spend on staffing, and often find themselves trapped in a vicious cycle, where more resources are consumed by picking up the pieces of poor care.

One of the most respected global voices on the quality of patient care is Dr Gary Kaplan, chief executive of the Virginia Mason hospital in Seattle. He told me very simply that 'the path to lower cost is the same as the path to safer care'.[19] While poor finances can lead to poor care, it is equally true that poor care leads to poor finances. Hospitals appear to have a choice of getting onto either a vicious or a virtuous cycle: allow your care to deteriorate, and more of your funding will be sucked up in putting things right, making less and less resources available to invest in improving patient care; but focus on reducing avoidable harm and death, and you free up those same resources to invest in ever safer, higher-quality care. Rather than safe care being something you just have to 'buy', it turns out to be far cheaper than the alternative.

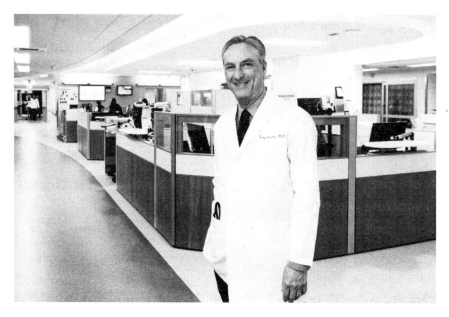

Dr Gary Kaplan at Virginia Mason Medical Center

Yet there is one apparent anomaly in the graph. Why do the worst-performing hospitals (ranked 'inadequate') seem to have better finances than those on the next level up (ranked 'requires improvement')? I don't know for sure, but suspect the reason is that the 'inadequate' hospitals have usually passed a tipping point: they have been put into what is called 'special measures' by the NHS, which means they can attract emergency financial support in order to turn things round quickly. For such hospitals, the vicious cycle has reached its denouement: poor management and poor clinical practice have turned a situation where funding is tight into a financial crisis. That in turn creates a culture of 'learned helplessness', in which all problems are blamed on a lack of resources and little effort is made to turn things round. Usually the only solution is to break the cycle with an injection of funds and a change of leadership.

———

Some people use the failures in NHS care to argue for a social insurance system, like that in Germany, Holland or Israel. While such systems often function effectively, they have one major characteristic that means they are unlikely to ever get public support in the UK: they allow wealthier people to pay top-ups for better insurance schemes. Such systems often claim that there is no difference in clinical care, just the comfort that surrounds it – but if a more expensive scheme allows you to choose any hospital (as they often do) when cheaper schemes do not, it is not really a defensible claim. The NHS, for all its problems, is regularly cited as the 'fairest' healthcare system in the world. It is recognised for giving people on low incomes better access to high-quality care – not just compared to the US, but compared to every other large European country as well. Equity of access is, of course, not the only priority for a healthcare system, but it is a prize we in Britain would never consent to losing.

In that context, it is ultimately a distraction to have a discussion about funding systems, when there is so much that can be done to improve the safety and quality of care within the system we have. Given our ageing population, we will of course end up paying more for the NHS through taxes, but Americans will see an even bigger rise in cost in their private insurance policies, as will Israelis and the Swiss in their social insurance premiums. It is entirely possible for the NHS to become one of the safest and highest quality healthcare systems without compromising its equitable foundations.

To do this, though, funding, staffing and a learning culture, as discussed in this first section, are the essential foundations of any change. But we also need to eliminate other barriers that get in the way of safe, high-quality care.

PART TWO

Culture Challenges

4

Targets

When I first met Deb Hazeldine, she told me she never wanted to be a campaigner. She was just a daughter who saw her mother die in the most appalling circumstances. She also happened to be very brave.

Her story started when Deb went into her local hospital to see her mum Ellen, who had been admitted after a fall. As soon as she walked into the ward, she heard a familiar voice screaming. She ran to where the noise was. She found her mother half on a commode and half on the floor, where she had been stuck for some time. Ellen grabbed her daughter's hand and implored her: 'Please don't let me die in here.'

Ellen was sixty-seven, in remission from bone cancer, and had been admitted to hospital for physiotherapy. She had worked as a dinner lady, always effervescent and the model of dignity. 'The kindest person you could ever meet,' said Deb.

But with the hospital focused on targets and financial controls, the elderly care ward was neglected and chaotic. Deb realised that if she didn't stick around, Ellen might not get fluids or food. Worse than that, just two weeks on, Ellen contracted two dangerous infections, C. diff and MRSA. C. diff is one of the most awful things to watch somebody have, Deb told me. It took away every scrap of dignity from a proud woman like Ellen.

This is because the symptoms are peculiarly horrific: without warning, faeces can be all over the floor, accompanied by a dreadful smell. Ellen would be sitting there silently sobbing, while Deb would spend a frantic ten minutes trying to find a nurse. Eventually, she would get down on her hands and knees with tissues and begin cleaning it up herself.

During her four months on the ward, Ellen was often covered in faeces, even under her nails; no one ever brushed her teeth or helped her to wash. Deb had to take in cleaning materials to make sure Ellen got even a basic standard of care.

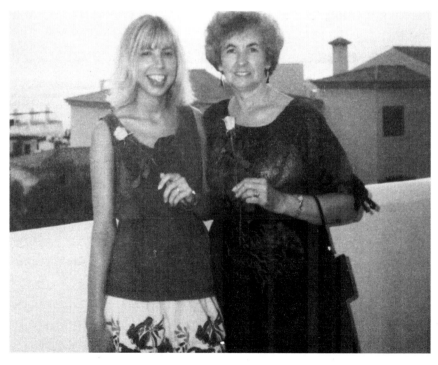

Deb Hazeldine and her mother, Ellen

Deb began to suspect that her mother would not survive in that environment. After visiting, she would leave the hospital sobbing and phone her father: 'She's going to die, Dad. They're going to kill her.'

At no point were the family told what C. diff was. Eventually, the physio told her that C. diff was a 'hospital-acquired infection'. Her worst suspicions were correct – the hospital had made her ill.

With no one to help her, Deb started researching C. diff. What she learned worried her even more: the guidelines said that patients should be cordoned off and visitors should wear protective aprons and gloves. But there was none of that, and Ellen was on an open ward with everyone else.

The lackadaisical attitude to infection control was demonstrated every time someone came round with a food menu, when all patients shared the same pen. Ellen would be sitting in bed covered in faeces and then use the pen, before it continued on its way to the next bed. Eventually, with no one to listen to her, Deb took in a box of Bic biros for Ellen to use so that she didn't pass on the infection.

Ellen also had two falls in the hospital. The hospital did X-rays which showed that she had fractured her back and spine, but because the results weren't referred to anyone nothing was done.

Complaining didn't work either, because of constant stonewalling. When Deb went in with her father one Sunday evening, there were no consultants around, so they were told to come back on Tuesday at 9 a.m. When they did, the same nurse denied outright that she had ever told them to return. The onus was always put back on the patients, who were told to work harder at their physio. It felt like Ellen mattered to no one at the hospital – just an elderly woman whose life was not worth saving.

There were, however, exceptions – and they kept Ellen and Deb going. The physiotherapist was wonderful. Near the beginning, he took Deb to one side and said: 'Get your mum the hell out of here.' He, too, knew that Ellen would die if she stayed for any length of time.

They never did get her out.

One day, Deb was standing with her father and brother in a corridor. Their consultant stopped and told them abruptly: 'Your mum is going to slip off and die.'

Forty-eight hours later, Ellen was dead.

But the injustices suffered by Deb and her family were far from over.

The undertaker and the embalmer phoned her to say that she couldn't view her mother. Because Ellen had so many hospital-borne infections, Deb was told her mother would have to be buried in a sealed body bag. She was in danger, said the undertaker, of contaminating the ground she went into.

The last few minutes Deb ever had with her mother were in the undertaker's, with Ellen's head protruding from a body bag.

At the same time, the hospital began to deny all knowledge of the infections and filled out forms saying that Ellen never had C. diff.

Deb raised her concern with the chief executive, who had been spending money on a new office suite. His principal worry was whether the hospital would be sued.

'Maybe you can put a price on your mum's life,' Deb told him, 'but I can't.'

Mid Staffs, the hospital where Ellen Linstead died, became the poster child for what can happen when NHS care goes wrong.

It was the first major crisis I had to deal with as Health Secretary. Although Ellen's story happened before my time, the public inquiry set up by my predecessor Andrew Lansley reported in February 2013, within a few months of my taking office.[1] It had been conducted by an eminent QC, Sir Robert Francis, with enormous integrity and compassion. In my first week in the job, I took home his earlier reports. What

I read surprised and troubled me deeply: was this really the NHS for which I was responsible?

Of course, it *wasn't* the NHS, or at least it wasn't a fair representation of it. At the same time as Ellen's story was happening, much excellent care was also being delivered – some of it in the same hospital. Indeed, the period between 2005 and 2009 was a period of record investment, record increases in doctor and nurse numbers and a big fall in waiting times.[2] It was also a period, ironically, of a big fall in hospital-acquired infections such as C. diff and MRSA – although clearly not on Ellen's ward.[3]

But Mid Staffs was not atypical, either. In many other unnoticed silos, equally poor care was carrying on.

I remember my first meeting with Professor Sir Norman Williams, the distinguished head of the Royal College of Surgeons and someone who was always deeply troubled by the high levels of harm in health-care. As he was leaving, he took me aside and said quietly: 'You need to understand, Jeremy, that this is not just about Mid Staffs. There are pockets of this problem all over the NHS.'

The Francis Inquiry revealed something even more disturbing than the existence of poor care at one hospital: it described a systemic failure by both the NHS and the Department of Health to pick up and deal with such problems.[4] Protecting the reputation of the NHS – and its political masters – had become more important than sorting out the care received by people like Ellen. It wasn't just that there were dangerous silos of bad practice: the NHS's own bureaucracy was conspiring to conceal it.

The impact of that cover-up culture was a dangerously distorted sense of reality among the staff working at Ellen's hospital. Robert Francis told me that, in their minds, cruel care had become 'normalised'. They assumed that care was like that everywhere in the NHS. Staff and management had little contact with better-run organisations and were operating in such a silo that no one – with a few brave exceptions – thought to raise concerns.

In the end, it was patients and their loved ones rather than anyone in authority who forced the NHS to tackle head on what was going on. Deb joined up with someone called Julie Bailey, who had also lost her mum, and formed a campaign group called Cure the NHS.[5] The first time I met Julie, she looked me straight in the eye, and said: 'You could be the one who changes this.' It was a challenge I have never forgotten.

But to stop such tragedies being repeated, I needed to understand why they had happened in the first place. How could such terrible care have become 'normalised' for the 3,000 people who worked at the trust? How could the national NHS bodies not have noticed? And when they did, why on earth did they take so long to sort things out?

So far, we have looked at the principal causes of avoidable harm and death – a failure to learn from mistakes, staffing shortfalls and inadequate resourcing. In this section, we will consider the factors that stop us from creating a positive learning culture based around the needs of patients. We start with Ellen's story, because it exemplifies what happens when healthcare organisations become over-focused on management targets and institutional goals at the expense of their own patients.

In the case of Mid Staffs, the Francis Inquiry made clear that concentrating on national targets led to managers deprioritising the safety and well-being of patients: 'This failure was in part the consequence of allowing a focus on reaching national access targets, achieving financial balance and seeking foundation trust status to be at the cost of delivering acceptable standards of care.'[6]

In other words, targets mattered more than patients.

Of course, targets are often designed to improve care for patients – not least by reducing how long they have to wait for care. So how is it that they can end up doing the opposite? To understand that, you need to talk to the people who deal with targets most in the NHS – the managers charged with delivering them. Most reluctantly agree that the NHS is a world leader in both the use and abuse of targets – although Stalin's tractor factories would have given it a good run for its money half a century ago. They appreciate the power of big targets to galvanise change in a way that can be of great benefit to patients – but they also know about the bureaucracy, gaming and poor patient care that can be an unintended consequence. I always felt that targets had an additional flaw: they focused the attention of managers upwards on their bosses rather than downwards on the patients in their care. David Nicholson described this as 'hitting the target and missing the point'.[7]

Much of the pressure created by targets comes from their simplicity. You either meet them or you don't – and that means they are of great interest to both the media and opposition parties in parliament. For that reason, they matter personally to a Secretary of State, who must explain publicly when they are not being met. Anyone holding that office thus ends up showing great interest in whether they are being met or not – and needs to be on top of the details behind them. The result is an extraordinarily bureaucratic command-and-control culture, starting right at the top.

To appreciate why this happens, let me explain in a bit more detail how it feels for a Secretary of State to be accountable for national performance targets. Tight budgets and workforce shortages, as discussed earlier, mean that waiting time targets for both emergency and elective care have become increasingly hard to meet. Indeed, I used to await their monthly publication with trepidation: a bad month meant shock headlines about 'longest ever waits' or 'worst ever NHS crisis'.[8]

I would invariably be summoned to parliament to be hauled over the coals, followed by an excruciating media round where I had to face the music about ever lengthening waits.

It also made for nervous Christmas holidays, because the NHS 'winter crisis' – when waiting times are always at their worst – generally started on the first working day after the New Year break. It was a date that could be predicted quite accurately, because it was when surgeries reopened and GPs sent a large number of their patients with problems stored up over the holidays straight to hospital. The hook for media interest generally came a week or so later, when the national data on missed targets was published.

I lost count of the number of times I apologised to patients for missed targets during a winter crisis. Apologising was the right thing to do – I was, after all, the politician responsible for the service. But it happened so often that I used to live in dread of someone putting together clips of all the times I had said sorry and use them to have a pop at me on social media, as happened with Nick Clegg's 'I'm sorry' video.

There is absolutely nothing wrong with putting politicians under pressure – indeed, in any healthy democracy it is essential to do so. But after a few years of frantically pulling levers from the centre to try and meet increasingly difficult targets, I started to ask myself what the impact of these all-dominating performance targets was on the culture of the whole system. Meeting Deb Hazeldine was the moment the scales finally fell from my eyes.

But before rejecting targets outright and considering how else to create discipline in a large system like the NHS, it is important to understand why and how they were introduced in the first place.

Coming from a business background myself, I knew perfectly well why targets can be a powerful management tool. In the publishing company I set up, there was barely a person in the two hundred-strong team that did not have a target of some sort. In a complex environment of multiple, sometimes conflicting priorities, they are a simple and effective way to focus attention on big-picture corporate objectives. As an entrepreneur, I used to ask myself, 'What are the one or two game changers we want to deliver in a year's time?' I would then make sure that nearly every employee had a target or objective that related to those key goals. They ensured we made big strides forward rather than just coasted along.

Targets are even more alluring to politicians. They allow prime ministers to make promises, fund them and hold both their ministers and public bodies to account for delivering them. Tony Blair, who introduced national targets for the NHS, wanted that accountability for a particular reason: he had poured huge amounts of extra resources into the NHS and was determined – rightly – to make sure there was a fair return for taxpayers. He correctly identified waiting times as a key issue, not just because they were a frustration for patients, but because making someone wait too long for treatment is clinically dangerous. The intention was that pressure on politicians and NHS leaders would translate into pressure on the system – and better outcomes for patients. Faced with the same circumstances, I would probably have done the same.

From Downing Street, Blair's NHS reforms were then implemented by highly able civil servants like Sir Michael Barber, someone who had moved to the private sector by the time I became Health Secretary but has now been contracted once again by the Department of Health to help set up a delivery plan for the Covid-19 backlog. He would regularly tell me that driving through change in a large organisation like the NHS is like wading through treacle. Without visible, public and national targets – and jobs at stake if they are missed – people remain stuck in their old ways and nothing changes.

Supporting Sir Michael's objectives on the front line were managers like David Nicholson, the NHS chief executive. I remember him once telling me why – despite the brickbats – politicians fall in love with being Health Secretary: 'It's the largest toy train set in Europe.' If there was someone in that huge, labyrinthine bureaucracy who 'got things done', it was him. Introducing targets and tweaking and enforcing them was often how that happened.

And they worked. Or so it seemed.

Waiting times fell dramatically for both elective and emergency care by the end of that decade.[9] A serious problem the NHS had faced for many years was finally brought under control. When subsequently the targets started to slip, the Health Secretary (me, by that stage) would vow 'never again' and resolve to get back to hitting them the following year. That response was no doubt exactly what their creators intended.

I would then sit in endless meetings with dedicated senior NHS managers like Pauline Philip, who was in charge of NHS emergency care. She knew her stuff, having run Luton and Dunstable Trust, which had the best-performing A & E in the country. Pauline is still doing the same job – and has not been able to enjoy a family Christmas for many years, because she is always getting the NHS ready for the first week of January. She is one of the unsung heroes of the NHS. Although we never got back to meeting A & E targets, I am sure that waiting times were shorter than they would otherwise have been because of our efforts.

Let's return to Ellen Linstead's story, because there is a very sad and cruel irony about her death. There was in fact a target to reduce the very illness – C. diff – that she became infected with. *And it was considered by the NHS to be a great success.* Alongside targets to reduce MRSA, it was introduced in the early 2000s following widely reported newspaper stories about dirty hospital wards. Not only did NHS managers set up a huge programme to reduce hospital-acquired infections, but NHS leaders like Sir Liam Donaldson, a formidable lifelong advocate for patient safety, persuaded the WHO to launch an international handwashing campaign – which later became critical in the battle against Covid-19.

Figure 4 shows the progress the NHS was making on those targets, impressive by any account.

So why, with the NHS so successful in bringing down infection rates, did Ellen go on to catch C. diff in the most horrible of circumstances?

The answer is that, although one or two targets can be highly effective, too many targets have the opposite effect. In other words, the effectiveness of targets is in inverse proportion to their quantity: if a

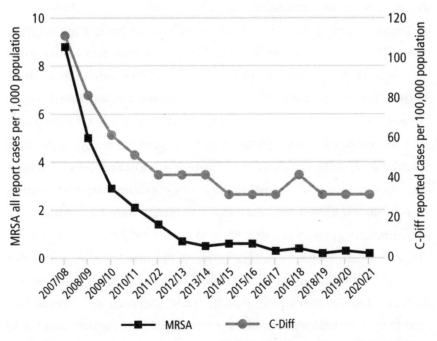

Fig. 4: Rate of MRSA and C. diff infections in England (Source: Public Health England[10])

hospital has 100 targets to follow, it may as well have none – because no one, however capable, can focus on 100 different objectives at the same time.

But that is exactly what we ask NHS managers to do. They have targets for A & E, for eighteen-week elective waiting times,[11] eight different cancer targets,[12] five new mental health waiting time targets,[13] the 'ambition' to halve gram-negative bloodstream infections such as E. coli by 2023–24,[14] targets on MRSA and C. diff, targets for vaccine coverage, including the flu vaccine every winter,[15] the aim to halve maternal and baby deaths and serious injuries by 2025[16] and the aim to eradicate HIV transmission by 2030,[17] among many others.

On top of which, a multiplicity of targets has led to a multiplicity of regulators.

Locally, there is the Clinical Commissioning Group (soon to be replaced with an 'Integrated Care Board') which contracts hospitals to provide care in its area. Nationally, there are NHS Improvement and NHS England, two giant organisations responsible for the NHS in England that are slowly being merged. Independent from them is the CQC, responsible for quality assessments. Then there are the professional regulators such as the GMC and the NMC, alongside the Royal Colleges who have the specific role of maintaining professional standards. Finally, there are other national regulators who also have the right to opine on health matters, such as the Health and Safety Executive (HSE) and the Competition and Markets Authority.

One manager told me that in an average year he has about a hundred different visits from regulators or national bodies – all with recommendations as to what needs changing. But no organisation and no manager can possibly process the actions from two external audits every single week. Some managers ignore them all – and tend not to last long. Others do what any human being would do and ask for guidance as to which targets 'really' matter. To which, at the time of Ellen Linstead's admission to Mid Staffs, the answer was straightforward: among all the priorities and targets, the ones that counted were A & E and elective care waiting times, and financial balance. Everything else – including the basic hygiene that could have saved Ellen's life – ended up being deprioritised.

There are other dangerous risks with a target culture.

Sometimes, when targets are transmitted through a large bureaucracy, people become oblivious to red lines that should never be breached in their pursuit. In healthcare, one of those red lines is that all care must continue in all circumstances to be safe. Many NHS managers understood that – which is why, even when the target culture reached its zenith, many hospitals continued to deliver excellent care.

But many did not, because often targets were passed down a chain of command without any attempt to explain the purpose behind them. One senior manager told me he visited Mid Staffs shortly after the scandal had broken and went into a ward where call-bells were ringing and patients shouting for attention – only to be ignored by a staff nurse frantically scribbling away at some paperwork. He asked her why. She explained she was busy completing care plans for newly admitted patients that had to be done before the end of the shift. She had been told that her paperwork was far more important than responding to cries for help from patients.

Targets can also foster a macho management style, with enormous pressure exerted from the centre onto managers to just 'deliver the numbers'. Not every aspect of good care can be quantified, so when a leader becomes over-focused on numbers it creates a disconnect between management priorities and clinical values. Communication between doctors and managers then breaks down, leading to highly dysfunctional organisations where both are contemptuous of each other. Clare Panniker, one of the most respected chief executives in the NHS, describes that as 'being about the number, not the patient'.

I should add that, although I personally ended up changing my view on targets, I was not wholly immune to their temptations. I introduced new targets on maternity safety,[18] dementia diagnosis rates[19] and E-coli infections.[20] I tried to be sparing in this, but in a way I, too, had fallen victim to the NHS management orthodoxy that I was simultaneously trying to change.

To counter some of the risks associated with national targets, the NHS now has an independent inspection system which is intended to provide a balanced judgement on all aspects of the quality of care provided.[21] It is run by the CQC, covers hospitals, GP surgeries and the care system, and aims to stop a single-minded focus on numbers at the expense of the quality of care. It is also designed to be an early warning system for future Mid Staffs-style crises. Thanks to the efforts of the first two chief inspectors of hospitals, Mike Richards and Ted Baker, the new system has worked well, with four million more patients being looked after in 'good' or 'outstanding'-rated hospitals to date.[22] I always hoped the new system would replace the targets regime rather than become an additional layer of bureaucratic accountability – and still hope it will.

Now, as we review the bureaucratic burdens on the system after the Covid-19 pandemic, it is surely the moment to take those reforms to their logical conclusion. We need incentives that drive up standards, but a decentralised inspection system such as we use for schools does that without the form-filling and other unintended consequences of national targets. As soon as you aggregate the performance of every NHS hospital and turn it into a single target for ministers, you end up hiring hundreds of people to monitor and enforce those targets – with local managers, regional managers, weekly data reporting and multiple accountability meetings. For people running hospitals it becomes more important to 'manage up' – take time pleasing the NHS England boss they report to – than look after the staff and patients in front of them. No other country in the world attempts to run its healthcare system by targets. We should ask ourselves why.

It is worth looking further at the model we use to raise standards in schools. Improving outcomes is as much of a priority in education as it is in healthcare – and we have seen huge progress in state schools over recent decades. The Ofsted inspection system is simple and offers an expert assessment of a school's performance that is easily understood by both staff and parents. We do not need to set the Education Secretary a target for the number of pupils expected to get good grades every year, nor do we have officials from the Department of Education performance-managing every head in the country. Rather, we measure the number of 'good' and 'outstanding' schools and track improvements in reading and maths through internationally recognised benchmarking exercises such as the PISA league tables.

It is worth asking what would happen if we *did* give the Education Secretary an annual 'target' for exam passes. He or she would be on the phone to the heads of schools that were underperforming – and rather than innovating to improve performance they would revert to obeying orders. Would pupils get a better education as a result? Absolutely not. That is why the appropriate benchmark for the Health Secretary is not meeting national targets but increasing the number of hospitals and surgeries offering high-quality and accessible care.

Removing national targets, however, is not the same as dispensing with clinical standards. We should continue to specify minimum levels of care, whether these concern the safety or quality of care, or the length of time it takes to access it. But rather than rely on a myriad of national bodies to blow the whistle when such standards are missed, usually stepping on each other's toes in the process, we should leave it to one regulator, the CQC, to identify the problem so that it gets sorted. As we have seen from the way schools are regulated, this is much simpler, much less bureaucratic and much more effective.

Although there were some signs that the government and the NHS were beginning to understand this, the pandemic saw the system fall back onto its fixation with targets as the only way of 'getting things done'.

It is true that some reporting burdens were put on hold and CQC inspections stopped.[23] But what did we do when we found we had less testing capacity than Germany or South Korea? Instead of copying their decentralised response, the government introduced a centralised contact-tracing system[24] run from call centres, and a new national target of testing 100,000 people a day.[25] As intended, the new target galvanised the system. Huge numbers of people were dragooned into getting tested. One of those happened to be my brother, who was in hospital for cancer treatment. He was suddenly told he would be tested for Covid-19 alongside every other inpatient – just two days before the 100,000 target was due to be hit.

The national testing target then became a classic example of what is now called Goodhart's Law:[26] the British economist Charles Goodhart argued that when a measure becomes a target it ceases to be a good measure and starts to distort outcomes and behaviour. So it proved: NHS laboratory managers were ordered to rush out meaningless antibody tests ahead of the deadline. The rules were changed so that postal tests counted as long as test kits had been dispatched – even if they had not been returned.

The effect of all the pressure was indeed a much-needed expansion of capacity. But at the same time other important factors, such as turnaround time – vital if someone needs to be isolated before they

92

can infect others – were ignored. When that became an issue, what was the government's response? To introduce another target.[27] So the cycle continued.

Ultimately, the government did (sort of) hit its testing target. But it also missed the point of the process: instead of a rigorous combination of prompt testing and efficient contact-tracing of potential carriers, we ended up with a national system that boasted big numbers but low effectiveness. The call centres charged with tracking down contacts only traced one non-household contact for every two confirmed infections; and at times only 20% of those asked to isolate actually did,[28] a far cry from the precision of test and trace processes in East Asia.

It is probably not realistic to expect a system to change deep-seated habits in an emergency. But as we put the pandemic behind us, the danger of re-embracing a flawed centralised culture looms large. Because of the interruptions to normal treatment, there are more than six million people on the official NHS operation waiting list, including just under half a million who have been waiting more than a year.[29] Many more are yet to come forward, so the real number is likely to be much higher. The government has recognised the scale of the challenge and in a way done the most difficult bit, raising taxes to address it through a new Health and Care Levy on national insurance.[30] But just like under Tony Blair two decades ago, will we once again inadvertently fall into the trap of putting in place a targets culture that turns patients into numbers? The NHS may have come a long way since then, but the early signs are that, in this area, it has not learned the lessons of history.

I considered scrapping targets many times. I probably introduced fewer than some of my predecessors. I also put in place the foundations of a much more balanced regulatory system with fewer unintended consequences. But I failed to reduce the number of conflicting priorities faced by NHS managers, with the result that running a hospital in Britain today remains one of the most difficult – and sometimes impossible – jobs in the country. Yet, unlike frontline doctors and nurses, NHS managers get very little thanks. I found myself leaving my job with enormous admiration for their good-humoured dedication.

Ultimately, the best argument for change is what happened to Deb Hazeldine's mother Ellen. Her story showed just how inhumane a large system can become if it loses focus on the people it is set up to serve. Deb and her fellow campaigner Julie Bailey paid a huge personal price for their campaigning: they both had to move out of Stafford as local people began to worry their campaign might lead to the closure of the local hospital. Julie ended up closing down her café and Deb had to cope with threats to dig up her mother's grave.

These two ordinary people did, though, achieve something extraordinary: they brought to the world's attention not just the existence of poor care but also, through the public inquiry that resulted, the cultural defects which meant that health provision, which should be supremely compassionate, instead became cruel and heartless.

5

Hierarchies

As illustrated by the story of United Airlines flight 173 in the first chapter, you never get far in a discussion about patient safety without hearing about airline safety. Sooner or later you also hear about Martin Bromiley, a pilot for a major airline who devotes much of his time campaigning for better safety in healthcare, following a terrible accident that happened to his wife Elaine.

Martin exudes zen-like calmness. His thoughtfulness and professionalism is what you would want from a captain if your plane was in an emergency. But he is also one of the most ethically driven people I have ever met, taking a one-third cut in his salary to give himself time to travel to hospitals up and down the country, to talk to them about how the culture in healthcare needs to change. I travelled with him on some of these visits, and learned from our many conversations that if you want to reduce avoidable harm and death in healthcare, eradicating the blame game is only the first step. You need a broader culture change, in which hidebound hierarchies are completely dismantled to allow people to work as a proper team.

Martin's story explains why – and, as with James Titcombe, his own professional background gave him insights that would otherwise have been missed in the course of the tragedy. Those insights illustrate another barrier that can get in the way of a positive learning culture: over-rigid hierarchies. We will examine the issue in detail in this chapter, in terms of the impact on both patient care and staff well-being, and then look at healthcare organisations in both the UK and abroad that have been successful in breaking down such hierarchies, and reaped enormous dividends.

Prior to his wife's accident, Martin had no interest in patient safety. He was happily married, with two young children, and getting on with his life. But his training as a pilot proved crucial: had he not had rigorous safety training, when his family suffered the tragedy of Elaine's death no lessons at all would have been learned. Ultimately that training led to huge changes, not just at Elaine's hospital but across the entire UK healthcare system.

It started when Elaine developed sinus problems. She went to see her GP, and routine surgery was recommended to clear them out. It was a simple procedure, so there was no cause for panic. She hoped to be home the same evening.

Martin took Elaine to hospital in the morning, where they booked into a private clinic next door to the nearby NHS hospital in Milton Keynes. They met the operating team for the normal pre-op introductions and everything seemed fine. Elaine was anaesthetised. Having seen her safely to the hospital, Martin left to take his two children home. Mum would be back to join them as soon as the procedure was over and the anaesthetic had worn off.

Later that morning he got a call from the doctor. The doctor was calm, but there was an edge of concern in his voice: there were problems, he said. Elaine wasn't waking up as expected. Martin should come to the hospital.

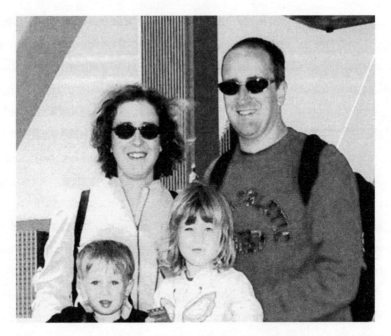

Elaine Bromiley with Martin and her two children

Martin dropped what he was doing and drove as fast as he could to the hospital. There, he was met by the anaesthetist and the ENT surgeon. At first, it wasn't obvious that the problem was serious. It sounded more like a normal complication: they had struggled to get air to Elaine once she'd been anaesthetised, so they had tried intubating her – putting a tube down her throat so she could breathe.

However, that didn't appear to be working, so they had transferred her to the intensive care unit next door.

Martin told me that as he hurried across to the ICU he had no idea about the true scale of what had happened. As he told me the story, I tried to picture how I would feel if it had been my own wife. You tend to close out the worst-case scenarios, because human beings have a basic need to cling on to hope. That was what was happening to Martin.

It didn't take long for that hope to be dashed.

As soon as he was through the doors of the ICU, the consultants broke the news to him. Elaine had been without oxygen for a while and the damage was severe. She had probably already suffered significant brain damage.

Struggling with shock, Martin was then plunged into the hellish helplessness of waiting. For the next few days, Elaine lay unconscious in a medically induced coma. Gradually it dawned on him that he might never speak to her again. If the worst happened, he wouldn't even have been able to say goodbye.

The agony of not knowing whether she would ever wake up was unbearable. And if she did, would she recognise him? In just a few hours, their lives had changed forever.

The days rolled on, and Elaine showed no signs of surfacing from the coma. Eventually, Martin was asked to make the hardest decision – to turn off the life support of a loved one. I shuddered as he told me.

Thirteen days after walking through the door of the hospital for a routine, low-risk operation, Elaine Bromiley was dead.

At first, Martin was too overcome with grief to begin to ask what had gone wrong.

During the time in intensive care, he had talked at length with some of the consultants. The answer from the surgeon was simple: this was an emergency that couldn't have been anticipated. They had done the right things. But as sometimes happens, things just didn't work out.

Martin initially accepted that analysis. As an airline pilot who knew the dangers of scapegoating people when things go wrong, he only had one request: no one should be blamed. He did, however, want lessons to be learned. Whenever an unexpected incident occurred in Martin's industry, people worked day and night to find out what had happened in order to prevent the same thing happening again. Martin assumed the same forensic process would happen now.

It did not.

The hospital politely explained to Martin that there would be no attempt to find out what lessons could be learned. There was no time and no point having an independent investigation – that's not the way things work. It was like telling him that 'stuff happens'. Although hospital staff were unfailingly polite and sympathetic, their defensive attitude was unyielding.

Coming from the very different culture of the aviation industry, with its eagerness to learn from every mistake, Martin couldn't understand why. How could somebody go into hospital and die unexpectedly with no questions being asked?

So Martin kept up the pressure and eventually persuaded the head of the clinic to get Elaine's case investigated independently. A leading anaesthetist came in and did a review.

Six months later, Martin gave evidence at Elaine's inquest.[1] With his background as a pilot used to safety protocols, he started asking questions about the way staff interacted with each other and the system they worked in – known in the airline industry as the 'human factors' at play during Elaine's care.

What he heard confirmed his worst suspicions. Something had gone very wrong with Elaine's care. Far from being 'one of those things', her death had been entirely preventable.

She had been given a thorough pre-op assessment. There were no particular problems. She was anaesthetised using a laryngeal mask to help her breathe, a perfectly normal procedure.

But then she turned blue. Her oxygenation fell. Four minutes in, it was below 40%. She became hypoxic.

So, six minutes in, the anaesthetist began a perfectly normal intubation procedure to get air into her lungs. At the same time the anaesthetist's assistant called for help. A few minutes later, the ENT surgeon came in. Following him was another anaesthetist, then another three nurses ready to help.

The three doctors gathered round Elaine and began trying to put the tube down her airway using different pieces of equipment, attempting to visualise what was going on with various scopes.

But the clock was ticking. Every second Elaine was starved of oxygen meant another second closer to disaster. They had to get her breathing again.

One of the nurses, on her own initiative, left the room to get a tracheostomy set which could be used to cut a small hole into her neck, a standard way to get oxygen into a patient when there is a blockage.

Another nurse phoned intensive care to get a bed. She came back to tell the consultants that one was available, but they looked at her quizzically, as if she was overreacting. Indeed, that nurse later told the inquest that she felt so firmly put in her place that she went back and cancelled the bed. Meanwhile, the first nurse returned with the tracheostomy set ready to use. The consultants ignored her too.

By this point, ten minutes had passed. Things were going downhill fast. With hindsight, we know they had reached a situation known as 'can't intubate, can't ventilate', a recognised emergency in the field of anaesthesia.

Even back in 2005 when this happened, there were protocols for what should be done. Surgical access with a tracheostomy was the most obvious course of action, and Elaine could probably still have been saved if they had acted fast at that point.

But a paralysis in their mindset had begun to take hold. Instead of rethinking their strategy, the three doctors remained fixated on trying to intubate – to the exclusion of any other option. Like Captain

McBroom not noticing the fuel gauge because he was trying to fix the landing gear, Elaine's doctors became so focused on their preferred solution that they completely lost track of time.

And this despite the fact that every minute without oxygen meant Elaine was closer to dying. The inquest heard that none of the doctors had a shared understanding about what was happening or what needed to happen. So none raised the alarm as Elaine slipped from consciousness.

Seeing this happen in front of them, the nursing staff wanted to speak out. In their hands was the equipment that could have saved Elaine's life. But the strict hierarchy in that operating theatre – along with the earlier rebuffs – stopped them from voicing their concerns. As one of them told the inquest: 'I didn't know how to broach the subject.' They could see what was needed, but they didn't think they would be listened to.

After twenty minutes, the consultants did manage to intubate. But it was too late. Twenty minutes at 40% oxygenation means the patient is, in effect, brain dead. The medical staff had been so fixated on one procedure that they had completely failed to ask themselves whether another approach might work better.

Even then, more mistakes were made.

Once they had succeeded in putting the tube down Elaine's throat, the doctors left her in the care of the recovery nurses and went on to operate on other patients. Their only acknowledgement of the situation was a suggestion that she might take longer to wake up.

As Martin read the independent report into Elaine's care it became clear that there had been numerous failings during Elaine's treatment: issues concerning situational awareness, prioritisation and decision-making, and failures caused by hierarchy and a lack of teamwork.

He realised that far from being 'one of those things' that can some-times happen, all the failures were down to those human factors – the way people had interacted. There was no piece of equipment missing that would have made any difference – in fact, the correct equipment had been brought in but not used. If the nurses had felt empowered to speak out, if the people in that operating theatre had functioned as a team... if, if, if those things had happened Elaine would probably be alive today. Martin understood this well from his experience as a pilot, where human factors and failings in non-technical skills are a direct cause of 75% of aviation accidents.[2]

Burdened with this new insight, Martin had to decide what to do. As he told me this, his calm voice softened.

This gentle, logical man was struggling to put his life back together. His priority was looking after his children and getting back to work. He had some tricky juggling to do – getting two young children to school every day is not easy if you are flying round the world. Then there was the grieving: he had lost not just his wife but the perfect family life they had built together.

Yet in the back of his mind were questions that wouldn't go away: how had it been allowed to happen? And how could he make sure it never happened again? Like so many of the people I have met, the only way he could find a sense of meaning in his life was to give Elaine some sort of legacy – a legacy that would stop the tragedy happening to someone else.

He found out there were lots of initiatives within the NHS ded-icated to patient safety and system improvement – but none were joined up. So he pulled together the specialists he knew and set up his own charity called the Clinical Human Factors Group, to pro-mote better understanding of human factors in healthcare safety improvement.[3]

Martin's charity has become an important champion of patient safety. He runs it on a shoestring and has been scrupulous in preserving the no-favours and no-strings ethos of the organisation. Thanks to his work, most hospitals now understand the importance of 'human factors thinking' for patient safety, and many surgeons across the country have heard of Martin and his story.

But Martin didn't just change the NHS. He also changed the thinking of the person in charge of it.

The first time I heard Martin was when he gave an interview on the *Today* programme. He was asked about my transparency agenda, and, rather frustratingly for me at the time, he said he would be concerned if it led to a blame culture. He was spot on in identifying, long before I did, the importance of getting the culture right.

After the disasters of Mid Staffs and Morecambe Bay, I had launched numerous patient safety and quality improvement initiatives. But I had steered away from anything as risky or nebulous as trying to change the 'culture'. I began to realise that this was wrong – the only lasting change in any organisation is cultural change. It was not simply the procedures in Elaine's operating theatre that were flawed, but a culture that meant the ears of mighty surgeons were closed to suggestions made by nurses.

How do you address such cultural dangers? In the airline industry, the human factors approach is deliberately structured to avoid the negativity of blaming the error on individual failing. Instead, the analysis includes the individual in the process of finding a solution. Because the error is depersonalised, the pilot who made it thus feels part of the solution and not part of the problem.

Of course, there are boundaries, and any pilot that behaves recklessly risks losing their licence. But the genius of human factors science is to provide a way to deal with the other type of mistake covered in 'just culture' – the ordinary errors that are inevitable in any field of life and that any of us could make just by dint of being human.

The result is a proper learning culture. And one of the most important lessons that can be learned about safety is the importance of harnessing the eyes and ears of every single member of a team, however junior, in identifying and heading off risks. Having had a culture every bit as macho as that in Elaine's operating theatre, the airline industry started to embrace a new, humbler learning culture. The results were spectacular.

Figure 5 shows the number of fatalities in the airline industry since the 1970s. It shows an extraordinary 75% decline in the number of passenger deaths, even briefly getting to nearly zero in 2017. Reducing deaths by three quarters is impressive enough, but becomes even more impressive when you consider the other line on the graph, which is the number of passengers flown in that period – a ninefold increase. In short, it has become massively safer to fly.

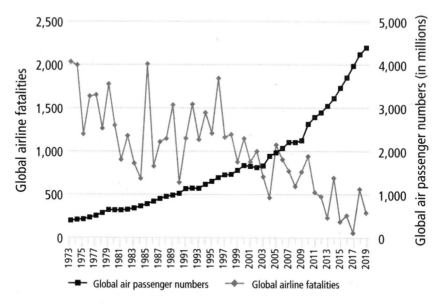

Fig. 5: Global air passenger numbers and fatalities 1973–2019 (Sources: World Bank[4] and Aviation Safety Network[5])

Indeed, by some measures it has become *80 times* safer to fly than in the 1970s – which may be the reason why so many more people are flying. In other words, the two lines on the graph are correlated. Even with the revolution in cheap flights, it has only been possible to increase the number of passengers at that rate because the industry has properly understood the way to improve safety.

What if we could change the safety culture in healthcare in the same way? Working with James Titcombe, I had understood the need to move away from a blame culture. But it was working with Martin that showed me what we needed to move *to* – a learning culture. So about halfway through my time as Health Secretary, I started talking about turning the NHS into the world's largest learning organisation. It never took off as a soundbite – and delivery proved even tougher.

Elaine Bromiley's story demonstrates the dangers of traditional hierarchies in medicine. The impact can be a failure to practise surgery as safely as possible. But it can also lead to the aggressive, bullying culture that sadly still exists today in some healthcare organisations. The impact on staff who have to cope in such an environment is profound.

I first met Helene Donnelly on a beautiful summer's day. She was expecting a child and full of excitement about the future. Somehow it felt a million miles away from the grim story I knew she was about to tell me about her time at Mid Staffs. But parliament was not sitting, so I had a bit more time to focus on what she was saying.

She described how one day, when she was working in A & E, a female patient in her mid-seventies arrived. A junior doctor asked Helene to help him get the woman out of her wheelchair and onto a trolley. Then they were approached by the Sister running the department, who looked at the lady and said, 'Oh god, it's you again…' Turning to the doctor, the Sister said, 'She doesn't need assessment. She was only here two days ago. She's just a naughty little monkey who hasn't been taking her laxatives. You need to get on and discharge her. Don't bother with her.'

The lady started crying. Hesitantly, she explained that she hadn't taken the laxatives because, without use of her legs, she was afraid of soiling herself if she couldn't get to the toilet in time. Helene and the doctor again tried to get her on the trolley to examine her. But the Sister wouldn't be overruled: 'No, we're not bothering,' she said. 'Just discharge her.'

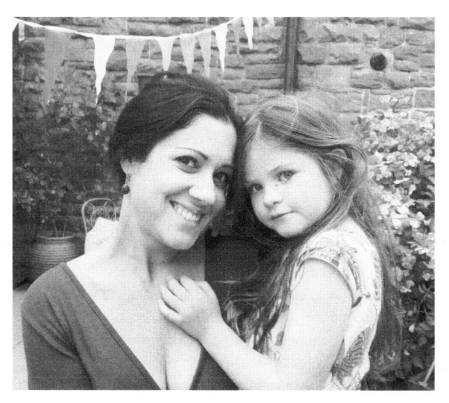

Nurse Helene Donnelly with her daughter Isobelle

Then Helene had to answer an emergency call, so she left the lady, who was wheeled off and placed in a waiting room to await transfer home. In the room, she started to vomit. Helene returned, got the lady a bowl and tried to comfort her. She called a doctor over and, now free of the Sister, asked him to examine her. But the lady had technically already been discharged, so the busy doctor just said she needed to go home. She was left waiting alone in the room, still vomiting. It took nearly eight hours before she was taken home.

The next morning, she was back again in an ambulance. She clasped Helene's arm and said: 'Am I going to die?' Helene reassured the lady as best she could. But it was too late. The lady lost consciousness. Soon after, she was indeed dead.

As we sat in my office, Helene's eyes welled up. My mind, though, was racing: these events had happened six years earlier. But was I so sure it wasn't happening now?

She reported the incident, but nothing happened.

That strengthened Helene's resolve, so when she was later asked to give a written report as to why there had been a series of breaches of the four-hour waiting time target, she decided to tell the truth about what had really been happening – namely that the two Sisters running the department had been openly telling staff members to lie about waiting times.

'For f***'s sake, just tell her to lie about it…' were the exact words she had heard. And wrote down.[6]

And lying was what her colleagues did. In fairness, that was probably not just because they were told to, but also because they may have believed that hitting the four-hour target could help the hospital become a Foundation Trust, thus securing extra resources.

But hierarchies are also bureaucracies. And no bureaucracy could ignore words that Helene had actually put on paper. So after her report was submitted, the two Sisters were suspended and an external investigation started.

Something else started too – threats and harassment. Walking down a corridor or going around the wards, Helene would hear whispers in the hallways: 'We know where you live…', 'Watch your back walking to the car. That car park can be very dark…'

According to Helene, the investigation was a sham, and soon the Sisters were reinstated. Helene was horrified, and the pressure on her mounted further. On one occasion she was even locked in a toilet cubicle and told to retract her statement. It was the last straw. Helene asked to be transferred.

But to her credit, her whistle-blowing had only just started.

She went on to give vital evidence to a Healthcare Commission inquiry, and became one of the most influential witnesses at the Francis Inquiry. When the scandal hit the headlines, she told me how she had listened to the then Health Secretary, Alan Johnson, say on the radio that what most worried him was that doctors and nurses had not spoken up. She shouted at the radio: 'But I did!'

She now speaks all over the country, giving advice to NHS organisations that want to change their culture. Her story – and Elaine Bromiley's – show in very different ways how culture can become poisoned by hierarchies that stop people speaking out when they have concerns about poor care. In Helene's case the bullying was overt, but in Elaine's case the invisible pressure on nurses in the operating theatre to toe the line was equally dangerous.

Despite the many wonders it performs, the medical world has protected those hierarchies for longer than most other fields.

In the business world, first names are common. Bill Gates is 'Bill' to everyone in Microsoft and Larry Page 'Larry' throughout Google. But – because it is a profession, because of respect for the long training involved, perhaps because of a long and distinguished history – there is much more deference in medicine. Doctors are still routinely referred to by their titles – 'Dr Smith' or (in the case of consultants) 'Mr Jones' – rather than by their first names. Such titles reinforce traditional hierarchies and create distance between people operating in the same team.

One reason that hierarchies persist in healthcare is that many assume they are necessary in safety-critical organisations. Everyone's role is defined, there is a clear chain of command and no arguing about who takes the final decision and who is ultimately responsible. What could be safer than a well-ordered hospital, where people know their job and follow orders? But in reality, overbearing hierarchies make patients less safe, not more, as Elaine Bromiley's story shows. Fear about speaking out stifled the very people who could have saved her life. Instead of ten pairs of eyes spotting what could go wrong, there was just one pair – that of the consultant in charge. If you want people lower down the ladder only to follow orders, then you stop them thinking for themselves. The safest hospitals make the safety and quality of care everyone's job – and in the process turn themselves into formidable self-improving organisations.

We need to scrap the outdated hierarchies in medicine that put the lives of patients at risk. And there is only one person who can ever dismantle a rigid and inflexible chain of command – the person at the top. We should therefore train all those in positions of responsibility – chief executives, clinical directors, even the surgeons in charge of an operating theatre – that the most effective way to minimise errors is to tap into the skills and observations of every single person in a team.

At the same time, we need to address the entrenched reasons why hierarchies have survived so long in medicine compared to other industries. One reason is that clinicians have been isolated from the flattening of hierarchies that has happened elsewhere, having existed in a vacuum for decades. Back in 1983, the Sainsbury's executive Roy Griffiths wrote a report for Margaret Thatcher which recommended breaking the stranglehold of 'vested interests' (senior consultants, in her view) on hospital management.[7] There then followed a sustained attempt to wrest management out of the hands of consultants into a professionally trained 'management cadre'. The results have been mixed: while some of the new manager class have gone on to be outstanding leaders, others found it very difficult to manage doctors who are reluctant to take orders from someone without clinical training. At the same time, the opportunity was missed to turn a generation of smart doctors into a generation of outstanding leaders.

Isolating clinicians – particularly senior doctors – from management responsibilities has meant that many of the trends that transformed leadership in other industries have passed them by, notably the power of collaborative, team-based leadership. The impact of such leadership was most succinctly summed up in the best-selling management book *Good to Great*, written by Jim Collins in 2001,[8] in which he quantifies the much greater success of low-ego, humbler American chief executives, when compared to their more charismatic peers.

The good news is that there are many extremely inspiring examples of clinical leadership in healthcare organisations where hierarchies have been dismantled as successfully as anywhere in the business world. Let's look at a couple of examples, one from the US and one from the UK.

Until 2021, Gary Kaplan led the internationally renowned Virginia Mason Health System, a non-profit hospital which is recognised as a global pioneer in promoting safer care through flatter hierarchies. He took his inspiration not from the flawed US health system but from Japan, where he became fascinated by the absence of hierarchy in Toyota car factories.

Every single worker on the Toyota production line has the right to 'stop the line' if they spot a defect. Doing this means that even the most junior worker can bring the whole factory to a halt. The effect is to focus everyone's mind on the quality of the cars being made, with the explicit ambition to produce zero-defect cars. 'We should be treating human beings as well as Toyota treats its cars,' Gary told me.

But four years after he became chief executive, disaster struck.

During an operation, a patient called Mary McClinton accidentally had antiseptic fluid injected into her brain. She died an agonising death over a two-week period.[9] Gary and his team believed in transparency, so took the courageous decision to publicise what had happened. They were predictably slated in the press – but knew they were right when it emerged that the same thing had happened in another Seattle hospital just two years earlier. Unlike them, that hospital had swept the incident under the carpet. Had they gone public, Mary McClinton might still be alive today.

Gary is a quiet, thoughtful man who has invested enormous time in flattening hierarchies at Virginia Mason. I visited him twice as Health Secretary, and always looked forward to long early-morning runs along the shore of Puget Sound on my visits. Each time I met Gary I was struck by how unlike a chief executive he looked. No grand office, the same white coat worn by all the other doctors, and as much humility as pride in his approach. He says changing culture takes time: having been chief executive for nearly twenty years, he had the chance to make changes that would be impossible in many other places. In the US, the average tenure of a hospital CEO is five years – and in the UK just three years.[10]

As a doctor, he is deeply proud of his profession. But Gary believes that the root problem is the way doctors have for centuries been put on pedestals by their patients, leading to a 'doctor knows best' paternalism that ultimately prevents the patient's needs coming first.

So in order to change the culture in Virginia Mason, he worked with his own doctors on a new 'compact'. The traditional deal for doctors, as he describes it, is entitlement to a job, legal protection and autonomy in exchange for their services. Everyone says that patients are the 'customer' in healthcare – but when Gary looked at hospitals with their waiting rooms, queues and hierarchies, it really felt to him like the doctor, not the patient, was the customer. Virginia Mason's new compact stressed teamwork, accountability and respect – on all sides.

He then set up a system of 'patient safety alerts' to mimic the 'stop the line' approach of Toyota factories. Everyone in the organisation was encouraged to report any safety concerns, however small. Initially, from the six thousand employees at Virginia Mason, he got around thirty 'patient safety alerts' every month. But now that has increased to no fewer than a thousand alerts every month – with every single one investigated to see what processes should be changed or improved. Just as Toyota's 'stop the line' methodology prevents faults in their cars moving downstream where they are more expensive to fix, Virginia Mason's patient safety alerts create prospective rather than retrospective quality assurance for patients. You stop the damage being done before it has happened rather than pick up the pieces afterwards.

On one occasion, a nurse from Virginia Mason called a doctor at home in the middle of the night to ask a question. The doctor bawled at the nurse: 'How dare you wake me in the middle of the night – just read the notes I left!' To which the nurse responded by issuing a patient safety alert. If doctors responded that way to night calls, how many other nurses would be deterred from making such calls in the future? The doctor was asked to apologise and retrain.

On another occasion, the hospital conducted a workshop to streamline the process of giving winter flu jabs to patients. A junior medical assistant pointed out that half of people carrying the flu virus have no symptoms. This could mean that apparently healthy doctors and nurses were transmitting the virus to their patients. 'Shouldn't everyone in hospital who has contact with patients be vaccinated?' she asked.

Gary readily agreed, and Virginia Mason decided to become one of the first hospitals in the US to make flu jabs mandatory for staff – an issue that has become of global interest more recently because exactly the same logic applies to Covid-19 vaccines. But when Gary raised the issue long before the pandemic, there followed an enormous battle with some staff. At one meeting, a young doctor stood up: 'I came to America for freedom. You cannot tell me what to put in my body.' At which point, a critical care doctor stood up and said, 'Never again will I take care of a patient that you may have infected.' The matter was settled.

Gary turned Virginia Mason into one of the most respected hospitals in the world for its patient-centred learning culture.[11] His job would have been much harder had he not been a doctor himself – but he showed me what is possible when a clinician is inspired to lead his colleagues. Unbeknown to him, he inspired another leader with a clinical background to follow a similar journey – this time much closer to home.

Western Sussex is an NHS hospital trust that has two hospitals, one in Chichester and the other in Worthing. The chief executive at the time of writing, Marianne Griffiths, is a vivacious nurse with an unshakeable sense of purpose. She was inspired by hearing Gary Kaplan give a speech on patient safety, and then worked with both Virginia Mason and another US organisation called ThedaCare to improve her own hospital's learning culture.

She described to me how she set out to make sure everyone in the organisation recognised that their 'true north' was to put patients first. Working closely with her medical director, George Findlay, she put in place a detailed improvement methodology based on Japanese 'kaizen' (continuous improvement) principles. She even has a 'kaizen room' on the top floor of Worthing Hospital. I remember visiting it and seeing thousands of Post-it notes stuck to the wall – the product of numerous brainstorms.

Marianne built perhaps the best learning culture I saw anywhere in the NHS. Key to her success was the way she involved staff in every change she wanted to make. 'I may set frameworks and objectives – but I never write the plans, that has to be done by the people who will implement them,' she told me.

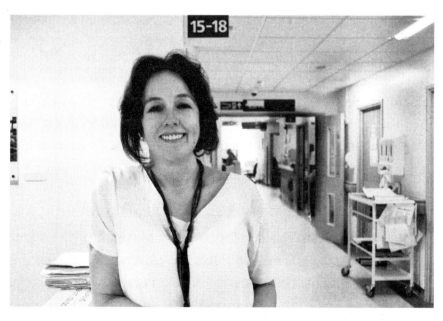

Dame Marianne Griffiths

Her modest manner also showed me something else: the safest and most successful hospitals in the NHS often had the most unlikely leaders. Rather than 'force of nature' types who bend people to their will, the more effective leaders tend to be more modest. As George Findlay describes it, it's leadership with 'big eyes, big ears and small mouth' – perhaps difficult medicine for a politician to swallow.

Marianne's hospital became the first acute trust in the NHS to get an 'outstanding' rating for safety[12] – and she has gone on since then to take over the main hospital in Brighton, which had been troubled for many years. Under Marianne's leadership, it has been transformed from an 'inadequate' rating to a 'good' one – with the biggest improvement in staff satisfaction in the country.[13] That happened because improving the safety and quality of care became not just Marianne's job but the responsibility of every single person working in her organisation.

I should finish by saying that exactly the same principles apply – although they are rarely followed – to government departments. Civil servants are discouraged from using first names with ministers, and generally stick strictly to 'Secretary of State' or 'Minister'. But just like hospital chief executives, government ministers need open and trusting relationships with their inner teams in which everyone feels empowered to speak out. Make a mistake and you can lose your job – very publicly – or become the butt of jokes around the world, as I discovered when I called my Chinese wife 'Japanese' (luckily she has a good sense of humour). This is doubly the case for elected politicians, because they are amateurs, not professionals, so the likelihood of getting things wrong is high.

I discovered how pervasive civil service hierarchy can be when making my first big policy decision as Health Secretary. After meeting my civil servants regularly to discuss setting up a new inspection regime for hospitals, I sensed resistance. The trouble was no one would say why.

They no doubt wanted to humour me, and rather hoped the Secretary of State's madcap idea would go away. Finally, it took the most senior civil servant in the whole department, Permanent Secretary Una O'Brien, to pluck up the courage and tell me the reason they were all so cold on the plan: 'We tried this before under Labour, and it didn't work.'

Rather than being angry, I was grateful. Una's intervention had saved me from a policy that would have failed. We drilled down to find out why the idea had not worked before, made improvements and ensured the new system worked. The result was a policy that went on to stand the test of time. But why did it take three months for my officials to tell me their reservations about the original plan? And how many other mistakes are made in government because civil servants are nervous about speaking truth to power?

What about the government organisation where you find the strictest and strongest hierarchies of all, namely the military? Obeying orders is part of its DNA. If you are going to ask someone to risk their life, many would argue you need the strongest possible chain of command. But do you? It turns out that even in the armed services much thought is given to how to make teams more effective by flattening hierarchies.

That is because in battle, too, over-rigid hierarchies make troops less effective, not more. In his book *Carnage and Culture*, Victor Davis Hanson argues that countries that embrace individuality and inventiveness have tended to win the big battles in history, whether it was the Greeks defeating the conscript Persian army at Thermopylae, Nelson disobeying orders at Trafalgar or the Americans defeating status-conscious Japanese admirals in the Battle of Midway.[14]

116

My father was a naval officer for most of his life, joining the Royal Naval College at Dartmouth aged thirteen, as happened in those days. Unbeknown to me while he was alive, he, too, was a strong believer in dismantling hierarchies. After he died, I read through some of the notes he had written during his time in the navy. 'Officers should be trained to disobey' was one of his observations. Nor, he said, should they be punished if the consequences of that disobedience were negative. People who show initiative and independence of spirit should be nurtured, because organisations that tap into the insights, ingenuity and inventiveness of their entire workforce will always be more effective than those that simply try to recruit brilliant people at the top.

In one place, though, such lessons are well and truly understood – the planes piloted by Martin Bromiley. Before he takes off, he introduces himself to every member of the crew as 'Martin', making sure everyone is comfortable with first names. The purpose is not to be chummy, but something more serious: he wants to remove any inhibitions his crew feel about speaking out, so that passenger safety becomes not just his job, but everyone's.

If Elaine's operating theatre had been run the same way, she would still be alive.

6

Litigation

In 1990, two bright young junior doctors at Peterborough District Hospital were attending to a fifteen-year-old boy with terminal cancer who was undergoing palliative chemotherapy. The boy needed two different injections, one intravenously and a second by lumbar puncture into the spine.

The intravenous drug was highly toxic – indeed fatal – if administered to the spine. But that was exactly what one of the doctors did, having been asked to do the operation on a child for the first time without any training. The other doctor, a senior house officer in general medicine, supervised the injection. He believed he was being asked to supervise the lumbar puncture but not the administration of the intravenous drug, with which he was unfamiliar. The mistake was fatal, and the patient died an agonising death some days later.

So what happened next?

You might think the most important priority would be to learn from what went wrong and make sure the mistake was never repeated. There might also have been some latitude granted for the fact that this was his first month practising as a doctor. Nor did he select the fatal injection himself, being handed it by someone else. But instead, the doctor was prosecuted and convicted of manslaughter. He and a colleague were given suspended jail terms, their budding careers in tatters.

Thankfully, in this case the convictions were ultimately overturned by the Court of Appeal.[1] But the whole case took more than two years, during which time the doctor suffered not only the remorse of having hastened a young teenager's death, but also intense worry about whether he would ever be able to practise medicine again. The very fact the case went to court sent shockwaves through the profession.

Even though in the end the legal system got it right, the shell-shocked doctor abandoned his ambition to become a surgeon and went into general practice. But there was something even worse: in its efforts to investigate a potential crime, the system completely missed the real crime, namely that while the legal process rumbled on *exactly the same error* was made in another NHS hospital – and another patient died. A system focused on blame managed to ignore the single most important priority – that tragedies should not be repeated. As we look at the barriers to a constructive learning culture, this chapter focuses on the impact of the law – on the behaviour of doctors and nurses, on securing justice for families who have been wronged, and on whether important lessons are learned for the future. We start with a story that shows the chilling effect of legal due process on the everyday behaviour of frontline clinicians.

In February 2011, a trainee doctor, Dr Hadiza Bawa-Garba, was responsible for the care of a six-year-old boy called Jack Adcock, who tragically died from sepsis at the Leicester Royal Infirmary.[2] She had recently returned from maternity leave and had an unblemished record.

The ward was extremely busy, and she made some mistakes. After assessing the child, she did not ask a consultant to review his case, although she did pass on his case notes. Nor did she make it clear that he should not be given a particular medicine, enalapril, which he had been taking because of another medical condition, but which would have been extremely dangerous for his condition at the time.

Nearly five years later, Bawa-Garba was found guilty of manslaughter by gross negligence and given a two-year suspended jail sentence.[3] She was then suspended from the medical register for a twelve-month period by the Medical Practitioners Tribunal Service, an independently operating part of the GMC. The chief executive of the GMC, acting on legal advice, decided that even suspending her from the register for a year was not sufficient, and appealed against the decision made by his own independently operating tribunal. In January 2018, this appeal was successful, and Bawa-Garba was permanently struck off the medical register.

Jack Adcock's parents understandably remain of the view that Bawa-Garba should never be allowed to practise again. But the context of those mistakes made many other doctors extremely concerned about the decision to prosecute. That day in January 2011, Bawa-Garba's rostered consultant was absent due to a teaching commitment. She did have access to another consultant, but was left as a trainee doctor in sole charge of the whole children's assessment unit. At the start of the shift, she had not been able to do a proper handover with the night staff because of a cardiac emergency, so she was under enormous pressure. There were also problems with the computer system, which delayed the blood test results. Should a trainee doctor, with a hitherto unblemished record, be struck off the register because of mistakes in such circumstances?

The case reminded me uncannily of the story of Captain McBroom losing his pilot's licence. Was Bawa-Garba going to become the NHS's Captain McBroom?

One of the most chilling effects of the case concerned her use of an electronic journal, which she kept updated as she was supposed to. Many doctors keep such e-portfolios to note down observations about their work, including detailing mistakes they have made and what they have learned. They then use such notes to demonstrate professional development when their qualifications come up for revalidation.

Bawa-Garba maintained her e-portfolio punctiliously. She also very honestly included her reflections on what went wrong with the child's care and volunteered her e-portfolio to the court. As it happens, it was not actually used in the court case by the prosecution, but the fact that it might have been terrified doctors up and down the country. Many said this would stop them making honest notes in the future. There was also great concern about the fact that a training form she had completed with her supervising consultant was used in court, even though she had not signed it off as an accurate reflection of what happened – many doctors were worried that private exchanges with consultants could end up being used against them in a future situation.

For my part, I worried that the learning culture I had been trying to promote could be holed below the waterline. For over five years as Health Secretary, I had tried to promote initiatives that reduced avoidable harm and death, starting with transparency and then – as my understanding progressed – focusing on the importance of a learning culture. I knew that a Secretary of State could launch a thousand initiatives, but in the end the law was the law. If doctors thought being open about mistakes would lead to them losing their jobs, that would be all that counted.

So I did something I had never done before.

There is a strong convention that Ministers of the Crown do not comment on ongoing legal cases. This is for a very sensible reason, namely to support the separation of powers between ministers and the courts. In this case the 'court' was actually a GMC tribunal – but the same principle applied. None the less, I decided to ignore that convention and go public with my concerns on the case.[4]

It generated a bemused reaction from many junior doctors, with whom I was not popular at the time, in the aftermath of the junior doctors' strike (the general reaction was 'Have I gone crazy if I find myself agreeing with Jeremy Hunt?'). But I wasn't seeking to influence the tribunal, nor did I. Rather, I wanted to send a signal to the medical workforce that, whatever happened in this case, I understood their concerns and was prepared to act on them.

In the end an appeal to the High Court overturned the striking-off. And in 2019 the tribunal reviewed the case and ruled that Bawa-Garba could return to practice after training and under certain conditions.[5] The decision was widely welcomed in the medical profession, although strongly criticised by Jack Adcock's parents. I commissioned Norman Williams to advise me on some important reforms, to try to prevent the situation arising again.[6] The GMC also made a significant public commitment that e-portfolios would never be used in 'fitness to practise' cases.

But the issue remains live for many doctors today. While Bawa-Garba regained her right to practise as a doctor, her manslaughter conviction stands. The fact that an error is fatal does not make it reckless – but the law leaves doctors and nurses fearful that they could be prosecuted for the kind of human errors that anyone could make. Legally, a court would have to decide such a mistake was 'truly exceptionally bad' to make a manslaughter conviction stand – but because there is no clear definition of what that means, the law is applied inconsistently across the country.

Dealing with such cases really needs a central police unit – such as happens with terrorism or child abuse – so that a trained team of investigators can develop the proper expertise to know when to proceed with an investigation. Instead, different police forces and coroners, often fiercely independent, take varying approaches, so that doctors and nurses are never quite sure where they stand. The problem is exacerbated by the inconsistent quality of 'expert witnesses' – so-called independent doctors who are called to give evidence at the trial. The result is little predictability as to which cases will end up with a conviction, and a blurring of the critical distinction between ordinary human error and reckless behaviour. That blurring has led to an increase in what is known as defensive medicine – medical advice or investigations carried out, not in the best interest of the patient, but because a doctor wants to reduce the risk of future litigation.

Any legal system should deliver justice and deter future wrongdoing. But in medicine it often achieves neither. For families seeking compensation, the legal process takes so long that they are often denied help at precisely the moment they need it most, such as in the early years of looking after a disabled child. For everyone else the hope that lessons are learned and spread throughout the system is often dashed, because the adversarial nature of a legal process prioritises individual blame rather than safety improvements.

The costs are also staggering. The NHS paid out £2.2 billion in 2020/21 in settlements for medical error, of which around a quarter was legal fees.[7] When I was Health Secretary, we settled about two multimillion-pound awards every week. The year 2020 saw the biggest ever single award of £37 million, to a family whose boy contracted a virus that led to catastrophic brain damage.[8] The fees paid every year to lawyers alone are so high that they could fund 7,000 more doctors or 18,000 more nurses.[9] One of the biggest trusts in the country, Barts, has four acute hospitals – yet still costs less to run than the annual cost of NHS litigation.[10] Maternity claims, accounting for nearly 60% of the total value,[11] now cost the NHS more than the entire cost of every maternity doctor and nurse in the country.[12] If we want to reduce harm in healthcare, this is surely a terrible use of resources.

The adversarial nature of legal due process also creates a defensiveness that is extremely distressing for patients and families.

In 2015, an eight-week-old baby called Benjamin Condon died unexpectedly from sepsis. His parents went to a meeting with doctors at the Bristol Royal Hospital for Children to discuss what had happened. They asked if they could record the meeting, to which the doctors agreed. But when Ben's parents left they accidentally left their phone behind – still recording. The doctors went on to say – in their absence – that the parents 'had a point', were 'absolutely right' and were not 'bolshy, misinformed parents'. Then they realised the phone was still recording and had a frantic conversation about whether it would be possible to delete that part of the recording before giving the phone back. One could be heard saying, 'I don't know how to do it without deleting the whole thing.'

The hospital was criticised for what happened in a subsequent investigation, and found to be at fault – but Ben's parents still had to go to the High Court to get the inquest verdict changed. Ben's father had to represent himself and use a barrister who was prepared to act pro bono, while the hospital employed an army of lawyers. The judge made it clear the inquest should be quashed before hearing any evidence. But why would a hospital decide to spend so much money on expensive barristers rather than safety improvements? And why, in that initial meeting, would two doctors feel so nervous about telling the truth to bereaved parents? Seven years after Benjamin died, there is still no agreement as to the precise circumstances that led to his death.

It would be wrong to say this is all the fault of lawyers. They can often be the only people a family can turn to in seeking the truth. In a flawed system, they can help to secure justice against the odds. But in general, is the law part of the solution or part of the problem?

One particular aspect of the law leaves families with children born with brain damage or another disability no choice but to go to court. Securing compensation is understandably very important for such families, who want to give their child the best possible future. But in England, no compensation is payable unless families can prove that injury was caused by a clinically negligent clinician or hospital. Because a finding of clinical negligence is very damaging to someone's professional reputation – and the reputation of the hospital where they work – a doctor, nurse or midwife will usually want to fight it. So from the outset, parents and doctors are pitted against each other in an adversarial process where the top priority is not learning from mistakes, but self-preservation.

Is there a better approach? The Nordic countries seem to have found a way both to improve safety and to reduce the spiralling costs of litigation. In Sweden, they have reduced serious incidents in maternity by half over the last decade and have very few court cases. The result is that they have been able to build a learning culture that has given them one of the best records in Europe on maternity safety. If the UK had the same mortality rates as Sweden, nearly 1,000 more babies would live every year – the equivalent of three babies' lives saved every day.[13] Sweden's stillbirth and neonatal mortality rate is lower than the UK's (3.1[14] and 1.4 per thousand births,[15] compared to 3.9 and 2.8[16]); and the proportion of inductions and Caesareans in Sweden is lower than in England (25% and 17.9%[17] versus 33%[18] and 29%[19]).

The Swedish system has four stages.[20] The first is a no-blame investigation involving families and clinicians to find out what happened and why. Families and clinicians often sit down together to fill in the claim forms for patient injuries – and because the claims are investigated in a non-adversarial way, conclusions are reached much more quickly, normally within six months. The second stage is to ask whether what happened was avoidable. This is much less toxic than in England, where the question is about clinical negligence. Even in Sweden, over half of compensation cases are rejected, because the events concerned are not deemed to be avoidable. But when they are accepted, the third stage kicks in, which is to work out how to support and promote learning from what went wrong. This is followed by the final stage, which is to support families so that they do not feel the need to litigate. Although they remain free to go to court at any stage, they rarely do, because to secure the same level of compensation they only need agreement that something went wrong.

Proving something is 'avoidable' is a lower bar than getting a court to agree that a doctor was clinically negligent. You might think that would make the Swedish system more expensive, because it covers many more instances. But in fact the opposite is the case. Because the Swedish system (and those that operate in Denmark, Norway and Finland, which are broadly similar) encourages a positive learning culture, they have a much better safety record, with many fewer instances of harm – and therefore far fewer court cases. Compensation levels are calculated solely on the basis of additional top-up costs needed by families in addition to state-provided care. When you combine this with a much lower level of serious incidents, the total proportion of health spend taken up by clinical negligence claims is around half that of England (see Table 3). A non-adversarial approach results in more learning and fewer tragedies.

System	Country	Population (2018, million)	Claims/100,000 (2018/19)	Cost per capita (£, 2018/19)	% GDP (2018/19)	% Health spending (2018/19)
Tort law	England	56	19	42.1	0.1%	2%
	Canada	37	2	4.1	0.01%	0.1%
	Australia	25	26	6.8	0.02%	0.2%
'Avoidable harm' compensation scheme	Sweden	10	167	5.0	0.01%	0.8%
	Denmark	6	183	-	-	-
'No-fault' compensation scheme	New Zealand	4.9	332	18.7	0.1%	1%

Table 3: Clinical negligence costs (Source: DHSC evidence to Health and Social Care Committee 2022[21])

New Zealand has gone even further than Sweden. In 2005, it introduced a no-fault compensation scheme, where payments are made simply on the basis of injury. Some worry that such a system would be very expensive for the NHS to introduce across the board, because it would end up paying compensation to many patients who do not make claims and currently receive nothing – but, as in the case of Sweden, the cost of litigation to the health system is around half of that to the NHS. Its supporters also say that it has encouraged clinicians to report mistakes they might not otherwise have reported, leading to much better data and learning as a result. A more limited example of the same approach has been taken in Japan, which since 2009 has restricted a no-fault approach to one of the most expensive types of claim, children born with cerebral palsy. Since then they have seen a 25% drop in children born with the condition and a drop in lawsuits.[22] The architect of the scheme, Professor Shin Ushiro of Kyushu University Hospital, says a major reason for this has been the reduction in conflict between clinicians and families. It is of course possible to improve learning and reduce cost within the confines of the current English legal system – as countries with similar systems such as Scotland, Canada and Australia have shown. But none of these have achieved the spectacular reductions in baby death rates that countries like Sweden have demonstrated are possible.

It would, however, be wrong to suggest that no progress has been made in trying to resolve some of these issues. I put in place an ambition to halve neonatal deaths, stillbirths, maternal deaths and severe injuries which was very ably led by leading obstetrician Matthew Jolly and chief midwife Jacqueline Dunkley-Bent, which contributed to neonatal deaths dropping by over a third and stillbirths by a quarter over the last decade.[23] I also set up a maternity scheme modelled on what happens in Sweden, to allow instant access to a settlement in maternity cases when the NHS knows a mistake has been made. It was designed to bring faster closure for families and prevent the frustration of long court processes.[24] To my frustration, it was not up and running before I left my role and ended up being cancelled, presumably on cost grounds.

Other initiatives have also made a difference. A system of independent investigations has been set up for every one of the 1,000 serious maternity incidents that happen every year.[25] They have been broadly welcomed as a big improvement on the much more variable and, according to the views of many families, less independent local reports done by trusts. These changes came on top of the 'duty of candour' introduced in the wake of the Francis Report into Mid Staffs. In response to the Bawa-Garba case, I also accepted a number of recommendations made by Norman Williams to try to make the application of gross negligence manslaughter law more consistent.[26] The Ministry of Justice committed to develop an agreed understanding of the application of gross negligence manslaughter law across the system and to improve the use of expert witnesses.

Taken together, these changes will help – and indeed have meant that England's baby death rate is lower than that in other parts of the United Kingdom. But if we are to achieve a fundamental improvement in our safety culture we need to go much further. Like Sweden and the other Nordic countries, or Japan for cerebral palsy cases, we should change the law to lower the bar at which compensation is paid from 'negligence' to 'avoidability', or simply the existence of injury at all. That way we would make it much easier for many families to claim compensation earlier, allowing learning to happen without the barriers created by a legal process. As in Sweden, the level of compensation awarded either by the courts or through an administrative system should be based on any costs likely to be incurred on top of NHS provision, not on the assumption that all the care will be delivered privately, as these days (unlike when the Damages Act 1996 was drafted) most families will continue to access the NHS for their child's needs.

At the same time, we should end the unfair anomaly of children from rich families getting larger payouts than those from poorer ones. Personal injury law tries to quantify individual loss, but what possible justification can there be for saying the child of a cleaner has less earnings potential than the child of a banker? To give different levels of award based on parental income contradicts the fundamental principle of equity upon which the NHS is built.

Finally, before any legal process is allowed to start, all participants should be obliged to go through mediation or an alternative dispute resolution mechanism. Many do ultimately attempt mediation, but only well into the process, when battle lines have been well and truly drawn. By insisting on it taking place within months, there is a much greater likelihood of it establishing the truth, in order that systems can be changed to prevent a repeat of the harm or death caused.

Such mediation needs to be part of a rapid, independent sequence of events that is automatically triggered after a tragedy such as a baby's death. The process should start with early notification to a national body that pays compensation when a preventable error has occurred; then it should involve an independently run investigation including both the hospital and the family; following that, there needs to be a rapid decision as to whether the incident was avoidable or negligent; any safety recommendations should be implemented immediately, both at the place the incident happened and elsewhere in the NHS; and finally, if there is still no agreement on compensation, there should be mediation or a binding use of an ombudsman before any litigation starts.

That would do much more than reduce the enormous litigation bill paid by the NHS. It would make sure that our top priority after a tragedy is learning and spreading best practice – something that is always the single biggest priority for people who have experienced a loss. There must be justice and fairness for any such families – but there also needs to be justice and fairness for other families for whom the same heartache could be avoided. Access to justice is not the same as access to litigation. As Karl Popper is reputed to have said, true ignorance is not the absence of knowledge but the refusal to acquire it. As we will see, if that can cause loss of life in normal times, in a pandemic the impact is magnified many times over.

7

Groupthink

The death toll mounted.

In a normal year, around 10,000 to 25,000 people die from flu and pneumonia in Britain.[1] A huge number.

But this was not winter flu. This was a pandemic. And getting on for half a million people had lost their lives.

The NHS was in a desperate state. Doctors and nurses were exhausted. Hospitals were full. Intensive care beds had run out. Many frontline staff had been struck down by the virus, some fatally. Those left behind were having to do what doctors dread most – make heartbreaking choices as to which patients to give the occasional spare bed to. Those turned away were almost certain to die – doctors were having to 'play God'.

In a nondescript government building in Victoria Street, I was shown into an airless ground floor meeting room. Around a long table were the key officials charged with managing the pandemic, including the Chief Medical Officer. Along the walls at the edge of the room sat more junior officials, known as the 'plus ones', there to record decisions and supply additional information to their senior colleagues round the table. There was a low murmur of private conversations and rustling papers which stopped as I called the meeting to order.

As always happens first, we all looked at the 'sitrep' – the situation report. It was a daily confidential briefing that gave the latest information on what was happening on the ground. Which hospitals were coping and which ones were falling over. Where the virus was spreading and how fast. How the other emergency services were coping. Anything new from the previous day was written in red. Despite the horrors we were dealing with, it was British calm professionalism at its best. I always wondered if that was a civil service legacy from the Second World War.

I had a 'chair's brief', which told me who to invite to speak at different points and what questions to ask. People made their points succinctly – no waffle at these meetings, unlike at so many others. I sat quietly, listening and absorbing the situation.

Then the Chief Medical Officer turned to me and asked me to make the most momentous decision I had ever made.

'Secretary of State, every intensive care bed requires four nurses. Those nurses can save more lives if they are redeployed to treat people in the community. Instead of saving one life between four of them, they can each save many more lives by giving out vital medicines to those in need. We are asking if you are prepared to close all our ICUs and switch off the ventilators.'

I froze. I was being asked, as Health Secretary, to end 4,000 lives in our hospitals in order to save many more outside.

It was a perfectly logical request. The greatest good for the greatest number. But something inside me just said 'No.'

Was it a lack of courage that would ultimately cost lives? Or a deeper instinct about what makes us human? In Britain, we traditionally revere pragmatism as the ultimate virtue and are nervous about allowing 'morality' to intrude into decision-making. But this time it was impossible to shut out one's values.

So I refused. I could not and would not do it.

'Stop the exercise,' I said. Because this was a simulation, not a real-life situation. 'We need to discuss why you are asking a government minister to kill a lot of people.'

This was the culmination of Operation Cygnus in 2016,[2] a pandemic flu preparation exercise that was held four years before the Covid-19 outbreak. It had taken place over three days and involved 950 officials from central and local government. Participants were asked to imagine they were in the seventh week of an H2N2 virus that had come from Thailand and affected 50% of the UK population, causing 400,000 deaths.

An enormous effort was expended on simulating the real-life decisions ministers would actually have to take. And we had uncovered an issue – namely that a minister (in this case, me) was not prepared to take a decision that would consciously and deliberately end the lives of a lot of patients. The need for better ways to do what is euphemistically called 'population triage' – having to decide which groups of people should live and which should die – was one of the major lessons from that exercise. The other was the need for emergency powers, which were then drafted and used rather sooner than anyone expected.[3] In implementing these recommendations, I was supported by Dame Sally Davies, the Chief Medical Officer at the time, who was always as fun to work with as she was formidable.

But for me this was not some theoretical exercise. A year earlier, I had chaired government COBRA emergency meetings when there was a real possibility of Ebola reaching the UK from West Africa. Britain had taken the lead in fighting the disease in Sierra Leone, and a huge cross-government effort was mobilised. One of the biggest risks was that the healthcare and aid workers we had despatched could bring the virus back to the UK. One, a nurse called Pauline Cafferkey, did just that. Thankfully, she survived after excellent treatment from a specialist team at the Royal Free Hospital.

Shortly afterwards, I hosted a meeting of leading health ministers to discuss global health security, a subject taken particularly seriously by the German Health Minister at that time, Hermann Gröhe. Whatever mistakes were made in the Covid-19 pandemic four years later, no one dismissed the issue lightly in the years that preceded it: in recent years, the NHS had dealt with swine flu and Ebola as well as the threat of SARS and MERS.

Thanks to this experience and regular practice exercises like Cygnus, when it came to pandemics the NHS was rated one of the best-prepared healthcare systems in the world.[4] Its centralised structures, so cumbersome in normal times, were good at reacting quickly in an emergency. Organisations that normally fiercely guarded their independence would drop everything and play as a single NHS team.

But nothing could prepare us – or anywhere else – for Covid-19. Since it is crucial for the NHS to learn from mistakes if we are to avoid errors and tragedies, just how did we shape up when faced with a disease affecting not one patient but millions?

The answer is: patchily. Not least because of groupthink about the risks we faced, groupthink I was guilty of myself. So let's look in more detail at the dangers of a consensus becoming so well established that no one wants to challenge it. Operation Cygnus, for all its organisational thoroughness, was affected by such groupthink. We will also see that an even more insidious example of the same issue costs millions of lives every year, even when we are not battling a pandemic.

But for the sake of balance I will start with some of the more effective elements of our national pandemic response.

Earlier, I talked about the importance of capacity – particularly staffing – if patients are to be treated safely. In a pandemic, physical capacity – in particular the number of hospital beds, intensive care beds and ventilators – is also critical. When that physical capacity runs out the situation can be devastating, even in well-resourced healthcare systems, as we saw in Northern Italy. In heartbreaking videos, doctors reported being told not to admit anyone over the age of sixty-five to hospital and to reserve ventilators for the young and fit. One doctor in Milan talked frankly about the dilemma this posed: 'It is a fact that we will have to choose [whom to treat] and this choice will be entrusted to individual operators on the ground who may find themselves having ethical problems.'[5]

Other countries showed, however, that capacity can be surged in a pandemic. In China, sixteen new field hospitals were built in Wuhan in a matter of weeks,[6] with stadiums and exhibition centres converted to 'Fangcang' or 'shelter' hospitals to look after up to 13,000 patients with mild Covid-19 symptoms. Many feared the NHS, after a decade of tight budgets, would not have the capacity to cope, but in the event it showed remarkable agility in building the Nightingale Hospital in East London in just two weeks.[7] The new hospital had capacity for 4,000 patients, equivalent to the number of beds in about ten NHS district hospitals. When it was opened by Prince Charles via video link, Colonel Ashleigh Boreham, commanding officer of the soldiers that helped in the construction, said: 'My grandfather was at the Somme, this is no different. I'm just at a different battle. It's the biggest job I've ever done, but you know what, I've spent twenty-seven years on a journey to this moment.'[8]

Similar, slightly smaller versions were opened in Bristol and Harrogate, and the vast majority of patients who needed ventilators or beds were found them. A high price was paid, however, by patients with other illnesses whose diagnosis was delayed or treatment interrupted: 330,000 fewer cancer referrals were made,[9] for example, and 34,000 fewer people started cancer treatment in England[10] – with tragic consequences for many families. How to maintain regular health services in a pandemic with 'clean' hospitals will be one of the major lessons to learn for future pandemics.

Britain's historic love affair with science led to another success story in our national response: the vaccine roll-out.

Following our experience in tackling the Ebola outbreak in West Africa in 2014–15, the crucial importance of more rapid vaccine development became clear. Under the leadership of Chris Whitty, at the time working for the Department for International Development, the UK Vaccine Network was set up, and British scientists like Sir Jeremy Farrar played a major role in founding a new global coalition, the Coalition for Epidemic Preparedness Innovations, funded by Bill Gates among others to help fund international research into vaccines. Early funding was given to the University of Oxford to find a vaccine for SARS/MERS that became the foundation of the most widely used vaccine globally, the Oxford/AstraZeneca vaccine. The UK then became the first country in the world to license and start distributing a clinically approved Covid-19 vaccine, starting with ninety-year-old Margaret Keenan in a hospital in Coventry.[11]

Now, back to groupthink: when Covid-19 arrived, a flawed consensus among the scientists advising many Western governments led much of Europe and the US into following a strategy more suited to pandemic flu than a virus with a longer period of asymptomatic transmission. In the UK that strategy was very public, with the four-part plan of 'contain, delay, research and mitigate'.[12] It sounded logical enough, until the implication became clear: the deprioritisation of community testing and isolation as soon as the virus started to spread beyond a few cases from overseas.

The result was that when the virus struck, there was an absolute conviction that we should follow a strategy best suited for pandemic flu.

It included deliberately stopping testing and isolating potential carriers (outside healthcare settings) as soon as community transmission was established. The consensus that this was the right policy was so strong that when Dr Jenny Harries, the Deputy Chief Medical Officer, was challenged publicly about why we were not following WHO advice to 'test, test, test', she replied:

> The clue for WHO is in its title. It is a World Health Organization and it is addressing all countries across the world with entirely different health infrastructures and particularly public health infrastructures. We have an extremely well-developed public health system in this country and in fact our public health teams actually train others abroad.[13]

Groupthink meant that we fatalistically believed that the virus was likely to spread to around 60% of the population at the initial pre-vaccine stage, despite evidence from China, Taiwan and South Korea that a combination of early border controls, localised lockdowns and strict testing/quarantining could contain it to less than 1%. By refusing to give up on containing the virus, South Korea ended up with no more than nine deaths on any one day in 2020:[14] had the UK followed the same strategy, there would have been fewer than a thousand deaths instead of more than 150,000. Korea, Taiwan and China also managed to avoid any national lockdown in that first year. After three lockdowns in 2020 and 2021, the UK lost nearly 10% of its GDP[15] compared to just 5% of GDP for South Korea.[16] Our economic bailouts therefore had to be correspondingly bigger.

There was further groupthink about the way the public would react to restrictions, with a widespread view that they would not accept more than six weeks of lockdown. So even when lockdown became an inevitability, it ended up being deeper and longer than it might have been because we waited to press 'go'.[17]

But even if, in those early stages, we were unwilling to learn from East Asia, we could have seen the dangers of such an approach from data on Spanish flu a century earlier.[18] Academics from MIT and the Federal Reserve Bank of New York looked at the economic impact of different approaches to locking down in different cities. They found that early and forceful measures, far from worsening the economic downturn, correlated with faster economic growth after the crisis. In other words, reducing peak mortality rates, or 'flattening the curve', didn't just protect health services and save lives – it also limited disruption to the economy.[19] As Gary Kaplan from Virginia Mason would say, 'The path to safer care is the path to lower cost'.

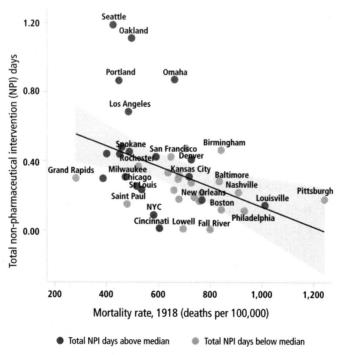

Fig. 6: Change in manufacturing employment in the US, 1914–19[20]

The impact on death rates was even more striking. Philadelphia had a 'spiked' death rate of more than 250 per 100,000 people because it took two weeks to stop public gatherings, including controversially giving permission for a city parade to go ahead. St Louis, on the other hand, brought in stringent measures straightaway and kept its 'flattened' death rate below sixty per 100,000.

Such mistakes were not deliberate or malicious, but they were preventable. Many of the key players at the time said subsequently that they deeply regretted not challenging the established consensus at the time. Matt Hancock, who was Health Secretary when Covid-19 broke out, told the Health and Social Care Committee in 2021:

> I was in a situation of not having hard evidence that a global scientific consensus of decades was wrong but having an instinct that it was. I bitterly regret that I did not overrule that scientific advice at the start and say that we should proceed on the basis that there is asymptomatic transmission until we know there is not, rather than the other way round. But when you are faced with a global consensus, and you do not have the evidence that you are right and the scientific consensus is wrong, it is hard to do that.[21]

Dominic Cummings, feared at the time as the most powerful man in the government after the Prime Minister, echoed similar sentiments when he said:

> I was incredibly frightened – I guess [that] is the word – about the consequences of me kind of pulling a massive emergency string and saying, 'The official plan is wrong, and it is going to kill everyone, and you've got to change path,' because what if I'm wrong? What if I persuade him [the Prime Minister] to change

tack and that is a disaster? Everyone is telling me that if we go down this alternative path, it is going to be five times worse in the winter, and what if that is the consequence?[22]

Governments, just like healthcare organisations, need to allow space for contrarians to challenge received wisdom.

Operation Cygnus, which I had led four years earlier, was also part of that groupthink. In our heads we knew there were many types of virus that could turn into a pandemic. But in our hearts, we believed that the one we were most likely to face was pandemic flu. As a result, by far the most resources were allocated to preparing for that particular type of virus. Cygnus was valuable and important – but being about flu, it managed to conclude without a single recommendation about testing capacity, which is much less relevant for flu because there is less asymptomatic transmission. It wasn't that we didn't do other exercises for different types of pandemic, just that they weren't prioritised. One in particular, Exercise Alice,[23] did look at Covid-19-style pandemics and issues around testing – but no ministers were involved, nor did any recommendations from it make it to their desks. One can only wonder how different history might have turned out if they had.

Ironically, having been so damaging to the early European and North American response to the pandemic, groupthink now appears to have taken hold in some of the same East Asian countries that were most successful in tackling the virus at the outset. They have remained wedded to a 'zero Covid' strategy, even though it is now clear that a phased return to normality through vaccines and natural immunity is more effective. The result is a continuation of border controls long beyond what is necessary when an effective vaccine plan is rolled out. They will ultimately pay a higher economic and social price as a result.

How do you avoid groupthink? Probably the simplest way is to increase transparency in decision-making, to allow assumptions to be more easily challenged by outsiders. Had the advice given to ministers by the scientific advisory committee SAGE been published, other UK scientists would have been able to point out the flaws in our approach more quickly. But for some time, the advice was kept secret – indeed, initially the government even refused to publish the names of SAGE members.

Groupthink is equally dangerous in more normal times – especially when it comes to the subject in hand, the prevention of harm and death. It has led to a consensus emerging over many years that a certain level of preventable death in healthcare systems is 'inevitable' – something that is fundamentally false. Because of such a flawed consensus, there has been a largely passive acceptance of around 2.6 million avoidable deaths globally every year. These occur simply because medical best practice has not been followed. In any other context such a high level of avoidable harm would be utterly unacceptable.

But in healthcare, because of groupthink, it has become normalised. This is partly because the number of non-preventable deaths is so high anyway. Around half of us die in hospital,[24] so as a result the average district general hospital has about 1,000 deaths a year, or eighty a month. We know that around three of those eighty deaths are preventable[25] – but which three? Shouldn't busy doctors, the argument goes, be spending their time looking after the patients that are alive and in front of them? Far easier, the logic continues, to accept the inevitability of some harm than embark on the complicated and messy business of trying to identify where mistakes have been made. The problem is that as soon as you do that it becomes less likely that lessons will be learned and more likely that the same mistake will be repeated. Groupthink about the inevitability of harm costs lives every single day – which is why it angers so many bereaved families.

Tackling such a dangerous way of thinking means not just winning the argument for resources, staffing and a learning culture, but also challenging that groupthink. Let us return to Covid-19 for a final example of the devastating consequences that occur when people who challenge consensus are punished rather than listened to.

Thirty-four-year-old Dr Li Wenliang was an ophthalmologist who worked in Wuhan. He loved food, especially Japanese food and hot pots. He posted regularly about his passion for food alongside other things on his mind on the social media platform Weibo. He was married with a son. His wife had another child on the way.

At the end of December 2019, he noticed that some patients had a worrying new virus which reminded him of SARS. He told a private WeChat group of old classmates about his concerns, advising them to wear protective clothing. His post went viral – to his surprise and shock, because they were only his initial thoughts. Four days later he was summoned to the Public Security Bureau, where he was told to sign a letter that accused him of 'making false comments' that 'severely disrupted the social order'.

Such was the strength of groupthink among officials about the paramount importance of protecting the reputation of the authorities that he ended up being one of eight people who were investigated for 'spreading rumours'. He was asked whether he would stop his illegal activities. Yes, he said, putting his thumbprint on the letter. He was asked whether he understood that if he carried on he would be punished. He gave that a thumbprint too.[26]

He carried on treating patients, but only wore protective clothing if they had symptoms. One of them was an old lady with a stall at Wuhan's wet market, where live and dead animals are sold side by side, including snakes, which are a popular delicacy. The presence of live and dead animals means that there is a lot of skinning in front of customers, which makes animal-to-human transmission easier – and although others believe the virus escaped from a laboratory, that may have been how he picked it up. After developing a cough, he sent his family away to stay with relatives as he didn't want to infect them. He checked into a hotel.[27]

Before he died, Dr Li became braver in his social media posts. 'A healthy society should have more than one voice,' he said in a video message that was watched by nearly two million people. Although most messages of support were deleted by the authorities, some were allowed to stay, because even they recognised the need for a valve for public anger. In the end the authorities apologised to him, something extraordinarily unusual in China.[28] After he died, they also said that he had not, in fact, disrupted public order and was a professional who fought bravely and made sacrifices. The policemen involved were disciplined.

But the damage was done.

China was, in fairness, faster in declaring Covid-19 than it was in declaring SARS two decades earlier. But it still took a whole month – perhaps longer – for it to tell the world what it knew. The Chinese scientist Lai Shengjie estimates that the number of people infected would have been reduced by two thirds if lockdown measures had been introduced just a week earlier in Wuhan.[29] We will never know how many lives would have been saved across the world if Dr Li had not been silenced.

PART THREE

Solutions

8

Transparency

I climbed out of my official car in a backstreet in Sheffield, and made my way to an office block next to the cathedral.

You never know quite what to expect on an NHS ministerial visit. This one was particularly unusual, because I was not visiting a hospital or GP surgery. Instead, I was coming to see an NHS patient, who was in the cathedral offices for a very specific reason. As a failed asylum seeker, he was not entitled to any benefits – nor could he work, because he didn't have a national insurance number. His only support came from the church, which is why he was next door to the cathedral.

The young man in question had schizophrenia and was being looked after by Professor Tim Kendall,[1] a deeply ethical and self-effacing psychiatrist whom I had got to know well. Tim was the clinician in charge of mental health policy for NHS England (a role he is still performing at the time of writing), so we worked together closely. Sheffield was where he practised.

Tim runs one of only a handful of mental health practices in the country for homeless people. Earlier in the day I had met one of his other clients, a middle-class man whose business had gone bust, causing him to lose both his home and his wife. He had turned to drink – and

Tim was picking up the pieces. The key to Tim's approach was to work closely with the city council, so that people's needs were addressed holistically: in this case the practical need for a job and home, alongside the medical need to deal with alcohol addiction.

But if the situation of that poor businessman felt desperate, this young man faced problems of an altogether different order. As we sat in the cathedral offices, he explained he was fleeing conflict in Niger. The authorities had not believed his account, so his asylum application had been rejected. But he didn't want to travel home – either because he was frightened of persecution or perhaps just because he knew he would never get back to the UK if he did. I didn't know the truth of the matter and was not there to make a judgement. But I did want to see what help we offered to someone who was homeless, unable to work and grappling with severe mental illness.

The only positive in his life, it turned out, was the NHS, which was providing him with help from one of its most senior psychiatrists.

Ironically, this failed asylum seeker was now looking at the Health Secretary who, more than any other, had tried to tackle 'health tourism'. I had always suspected that many people from abroad were coming to the UK to benefit from NHS care they were not entitled to. As a result, I had a number of battles with parts of the NHS establishment who either did not believe it was happening, or – even if they did – believed it was wrong to tackle it, on the basis that the NHS should be there for anyone who turned up needing help.

Now I found myself feeling rather different.

It was perfectly legal for him to be an NHS patient, even though he had never contributed to the NHS by paying taxes (although the rules said he would have to pay for any hospital care). And, rather to my surprise, I found myself feeling proud to be in one of the few countries in the world where a homeless failed asylum seeker could access mental health care, free of charge, from a top psychiatrist. Was that consistent with my earlier instincts? Probably not, but sometimes experience collides with belief.

There was, however, something problematic about Tim's practice in Sheffield that was nothing to do with my views on health tourism.

The work he was doing with homeless people was groundbreaking, really sorting out problems and putting people back on their feet. It was probably saving the state lots of money too. But despite its evident success, there were only a handful of similar services across the country. Few people knew what Tim was up to, because he was working in a silo that was cut off from the rest of the system.

One of the biggest challenges I was facing was the huge number of silos in the world's fifth largest organisation. Bill Clinton once said that politics is like working in a graveyard – there are lots of people underneath you, but they are not necessarily listening.[2] It often felt like that being responsible for an organisation of 1.4 million employees. Figuring out the safest and most effective way to look after a patient was usually the easy bit: getting that best practice adopted across a large system was a thousand times harder.

But if the NHS's internal barriers were frustrating, they were nothing compared to the solid walls that went up when it wanted to shut out outsiders. I found that out from a couple who came to see me in my office just a few months after I had become Health Secretary.

Scott Morrish is a photographer, and his wife Sue a graphic designer. They live in Devon, and both are straightforward and decent as well as being devoted parents. Which made the story of the death of their three-year-old son Sam even more heartbreaking. Sam had sepsis. Unfortunately, it was not spotted by the phone helpline his parents called, nor by his GP. It was not even spotted at his local hospital when he was rushed into A & E – but not screened for sepsis on arrival. As a result, he was not given the antibiotics that could have saved him until it was too late. As a father myself, I felt a chill down my spine when Scott and Sue told me they had to listen to the words every parent dreads: 'I'm sorry, there is nothing more that can be done.'

But what happened next was equally troubling.

Sam's parents were told by the hospital that Sam had suffered from an incredibly rare form of flu alongside an infection, so he could not have been saved. Devastated, they grieved for six months before questions about Sam's care began to niggle. Some of the descriptions of his condition were incorrectly recorded. At key moments in his care, they found out they had been speaking to people without medical qualifications. The antibiotics Sam was prescribed weren't given to him for three critical hours. No one mentioned sepsis.

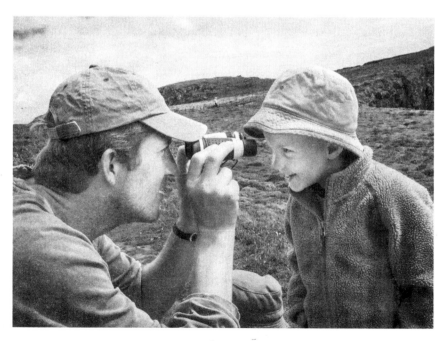

Scott and Sam Morrish

When they tried to raise these concerns, they experienced a brick wall. The shutters came down. No one was prepared to meet them. Scott told me, like so many other families did subsequently: 'I never wanted anyone to be fired. I wanted them all to stay, improve and learn [...] so that other tragedies could be avoided. But the system doesn't understand that. It only ever saw me as a problem.'

When it came to that system, I knew the buck stopped with me.

I happen to know that the hospital concerned subsequently took the lessons of Sam's death to heart – but the bureaucratic defensiveness Scott and Sue described still rears its head today. As I listened to them in my comfortable ministerial office, I sensed I was being judged: tea and sympathy was fine – but what was going to change? How was I going to transform a closed culture full of internal and external walls into an open one, where people are hungry to learn from mistakes and embrace the most effective way of doing things?

I didn't have the answer at that meeting. But as we have seen, transparency is the vital first step. In this section we will be looking at the most effective solutions for reducing avoidable harm and death, and so we start with that first step: what are the best strategies for embedding an open and transparent culture? How can we prioritise the sharing of best practice – such as at Tim Kendall's homelessness clinic – alongside being open when mistakes are made, such as with Sam Morrish?

Finding out the truth when something has gone wrong can be difficult, as we have seen many times. Much easier, it turns out, is collecting and sharing data about all the care a doctor, or team of doctors, delivers. When you do that, however, the results are no less shocking, because they reveal that the quality of care across the NHS is much more variable than most imagine.

That variation in the quality of care was something I came to understand principally through the work of a surgeon called Tim

Briggs. Tim is a professor at the Royal National Orthopaedic Hospital in north-west London. His passion, as an orthopaedic surgeon of thirty years, is improving outcomes for all patients by reducing unwarranted variation and complications such as infection rates.

He knew that if a prosthetic joint such as a hip or knee becomes infected after surgery it can be devastating for a patient. To get rid of the infection requires a series of follow-up procedures, often involving replacing the new prosthetic knee or hip in a succession of operations. During this time the patient, despite being immobile, has to find a way to get to hospital regularly. Even after those repeated operations there is no guarantee of success, and sometimes the process ends up with an amputation.

To avoid this, orthopaedic surgeons go to enormous trouble to avoid infections happening. As well as more obvious measures like hand hygiene, operating theatres have special air filtration systems which drive purified air onto the patient in the middle of the theatre to avoid the risk of airborne infections.

The natural thing to do for a surgeon like Tim would have been to focus on finding ways to reduce infections in his own practice and then encourage others to adopt any new techniques he discovered, perhaps by writing a paper for the Royal College of Surgeons or the *British Medical Journal*.

But he went a step further. He decided to try to quantify the problem – and not just for his hospital. He set about seeing if he could measure the scale of the issue for the whole of the NHS in England and then use the data to drive improvements in the quality of surgery throughout the system. He then banged on the door of ministers (including me) and NHS top brass to secure the support and resources he needed to complete his mission.

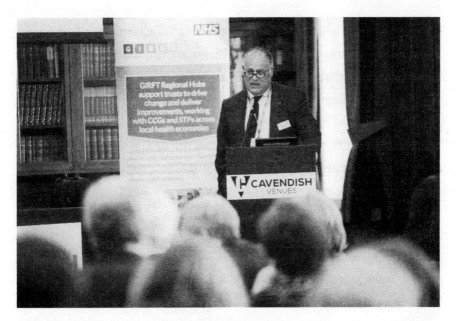

Professor Tim Briggs

After he had secured the support he needed, he set about cajoling his orthopaedic surgeon colleagues up and down the country to share and use data to improve their practice. Key to his success was giving his colleagues confidence that their data was not going to be published. It was a 'surgeon to surgeon' process, purely and simply designed to improve clinical practice.

Slowly, he won the trust of his orthopaedic colleagues, and over a period of two years was able to visit every hospital trust in England as well as many in Scotland, Wales and Northern Ireland. He tracked over 150 different metrics including infection rates.

The results that came back were extraordinary.

It was then that the scale of variation become shockingly apparent.

The best orthopaedic infection rate recorded in the NHS was around one in five hundred patients. But the worst – to his surprise – was as high as one in twenty patients. One major city had, quite near each other, both a hospital with one of the best infection rates and a hospital with an infection rate twenty times higher. Residents there were using two neighbouring hospitals on the assumption that the quality of care was similar – but one was about the safest in the NHS and the other one of the least safe. What made it worse was that neither had any idea of the *twentyfold* difference in the quality of care they were delivering compared to their neighbour.

	No. of orthopaedic processes reported	% with infections – initial patient spell	% with infections – initial patient spell + readmission
Trust 1	349	1.43%	1.43%
Trust 2	116	1.72%	1.72%
Trust 3	809	1.11%	2.47%
Trust 4	685	0.58%	0.73%
Trust 5	156	3.85%	4.49%
Trust 6	2657	0.68%	1.05%
Trust 7	454	0.00%	0.22%
Trust 8	544	1.47%	2.21%
Trust 9	521	0.00%	0.19%

Table 4: Difference between nine trusts in infection rates for hip and knee replacement (Source: Getting it Right First Time Programme[3])

This variation was linked to an equivalent variation in cost. While the standard cost of replacing a hip or knee in the NHS is around £6,000,[4] the cost of cleaning up a complication can rise to £100,000[5] because of the additional GP and hospital appointments, repeated surgery, long-term antibiotics and hospitalisation.

But even that additional cost is dwarfed by the litigation that inevitably follows the failures in surgery. Negligence claims at the time were rising in orthopaedic surgery, with more litigation than any other specialty and the third-highest total costs. So, using the data he had collected, Tim worked out the additional cost of litigation claims for each hospital. The average extra cost was £54 per procedure. But in the best hospitals there was no additional surcharge – while for others it was as much as £151 per procedure. This data, too, he shared with every hospital trust.

When surgeons saw their personal performance data, if the result was disappointing their first reaction was – perhaps unsurprisingly – to question the quality of the data. 'Tim, your data's rubbish,' or something similar, would be the response. But after sharing as many as twelve different data sets telling the same story, the data became impossible to doubt.

The effect of this transparency on performance was electric.

Surgeons with the higher infection rates wanted to understand why. Without any central instructions from the Department of Health or the NHS, clinical standards started to improve.

Following the introduction of Tim's 'Getting it Right First Time' programme (GIRFT), the number of hip operations that had to be redone because the first operation was not successful fell every year. Tim believes that the reduction in orthopaedic infection rates over the first five years of the programme has prevented 60,000 patients getting an infection – or around 1,000 fewer infections *every month*. Each infection avoided doesn't just save on the cost of follow-up surgery or potential litigation – it saves the patient enormous stress and pain.[6]

Litigation costs also started to fall dramatically.

In the first four years of the programme, there were year-on-year drops in the litigation bill, as well as drops in the total number of claims against orthopaedic surgeons.[7] Orthopaedic surgery ceased being the most litigated specialty. The NHS saved around £64 million, as the number of revision procedures and associated hospital stays was reduced. Further savings occurred because fewer replacement hips or knees needed to be sourced.

Clinical practice also changed. Many surgeons used to enjoy doing the occasional 'complex' procedure. It was professionally interesting and no doubt educational. But the data showed clearly that complex procedures done 'occasionally' were far more likely to lead to complications and revisions. After Tim's data was shared, 'occasional complex surgery' reduced significantly. Such jobs were passed on to surgeons who specialise in them – further reducing the risk to patients.

This was not transparency imposed from above. It was a much more subtle and intelligent transparency that went with the grain of every doctor's desire to do the best for their patients. Collecting and sharing data was the fastest and most effective way of breaking down closed silos and spreading best practice – because it played to the unusual combination of competitiveness and altruism that is innate to most doctors. Ironically it was that same NHS bureaucracy, such a nightmare for Scott and Sue Morrish, which made it possible.

The GIRFT programme has now expanded to every surgical and medical specialty. Tim has around sixty-six clinical directors working for him across forty specialties, and is even doing pilots in community care and general practice.[8] The scheme has expanded to independent sector hospitals in the UK. It has also expanded internationally,[9] and is being considered in many other countries as well as having been adopted in Queensland, Australia.

One offshoot of the plan has been the extraction not just of unit-level data but of surgeon-level data. Under a sister programme called the National Consultant Information Programme[10] led by Norman Williams, GIRFT is now starting to share data with surgeons regarding not just their unit's performance, but their individual performance as well. This of course already happens in many good hospitals around the world – but what makes it unique is the way this data is shared both inside a hospital and throughout an entire health system.

Of course, there is no point sharing data unless it leads to improvements in clinical practice. And perhaps the best example of how to use data to follow through with such improvements comes from another Tim, Tim Draycott, who has used the same principles of data transparency to transform the safety of maternity services.

Tim now runs the maternity unit at Southmead Hospital in Bristol. As a young registrar there, he once tried to deliver a baby whose shoulders got stuck inside the mother's womb. The child's head had emerged, but the rest of the body refused to shift. He finally got the baby out with the help of a senior colleague, but the child's shoulder was damaged. Tim realised that although he had known what to do in theory, he had blanked for two or three critical minutes in the heat of an emergency.

So he started to develop techniques that radically reduced the number of babies injured during birth. As he described it to me, he wanted to make 'the right way the easy way'. The NICE maternity guidelines had 160 pages, but it was totally impractical to expect someone to plough through them in an emergency. Instead, Tim gave his colleagues a simple cardboard box which contained all the equipment necessary for particular types of emergency. Each box also included a clear flow chart of instructions, known as the 'algorithm', and was kept on hand so that it could be grabbed immediately if needed.

Soon the improvements started happening. Tim began to realise he was on to something when he was criticised by another consultant for the small number of hypoxic or oxygen-starved children he was sending through for emergency care. The consultant assumed the reason was that the children were dying before they could get access to life-saving care. But the real reason was the opposite: by making his surgery safer, Tim had reduced the number of hypoxic children born in Southmead to one third of the national average.

The maternity unit where Tim works is now one of the safest in Europe, and by sharing performance data among his colleagues in other hospitals he has encouraged maternity units to use his 'PROMPT' system in over seventy countries worldwide. He reckons that when you share data, around a third of hospitals with below-average performance data self-correct. The others need help to improve – which now happens with the national programme led by leading obstetrician Matthew Jolly and chief midwife Jacqueline Dunkley-Bent.[11] Thanks to their efforts, as we saw earlier, baby deaths in the NHS in England have reduced by over a third over the last decade.[12]

It is worth pointing out that the two Tims were not the first NHS consultants to champion the power of transparency. A decade earlier, Bruce Keogh had pioneered the sharing of data by heart surgeons following the Bristol Royal Hospital for Children scandal of the 1990s. It took him over a decade to get agreement to publish survival rates for individual heart surgeons – but the result, once again, was a dramatic improvement in the safety and success of cardiac surgery. Norman Williams was another transparency pioneer as head of the Royal College of Surgeons, when he bravely championed the publication of outcome data by individual surgeons, against the wishes of many in his own profession.[13]

But why should it take such an effort on the part of inspiring individuals to break open a closed culture? Surely it should be a matter of course for professionals and units performing safety-critical procedures to share and learn from their performance data. Indeed, *not* sharing performance data is the real crime, given the known dangers of operating in a silo. The problem is that there is always professional resistance to transparency – indeed, although Tim Briggs's programme is going from strength to strength, other initiatives to publish surgery outcome data have stalled, quietly removed from the NHS website for 'cost reasons'. If we want an open culture, transparency should be the default.

But it is not without risks – and such risks should be managed carefully.

Any data that is published must be accurate, because mistakes can have terrible consequences. When the first set of data on vascular surgery performance was published in 2013, it wrongly identified an unfortunate surgeon in Portsmouth as having some of the highest mortality rates in the country – even though he had not practised for many years.[14] Assembling good-quality data needs collaboration from clinicians, which often means making a commitment that individual performance data will not be made public. That can be a price worth paying.

There is also the risk that knowing outcomes are being measured can lead to inappropriate distortions in clinical decision-making. The heart surgeon Samer Nashef shows how this happens in his very thoughtful book *The Naked Surgeon*,[15] which quotes an anonymous survey of UK heart surgeons, asking whether they had given potentially unnecessary heart surgery to a patient in order to shift the categorisation of the operation from lower to higher risk, thus improving their reported personal outcomes. Of 115 surgeons surveyed, just over 10% said they had done this, but more than half said they were aware of other surgeons doing it.

But as Nashef also points out, other studies show the opposite effect: an increase in the safety of care caused simply by someone knowing their outcomes are being measured. This is known as the Hawthorne effect, after studies done at the Hawthorne Works, a US electrical goods factory, in the 1920s. Everyone is human – and sensitive to their own reputation. Nashef observed the same phenomenon when he introduced the EuroSCORE measurement system for heart surgery outcomes. He also pioneered the use of teams to review and take responsibility for higher-risk surgery, so that individual surgeons were not tempted to adjust clinical advice if it might affect their personal outcome rates.

Transparency can be as painful for institutions as for individuals. Many worried about the impact on staff morale when a new and independent rating system for hospitals put thirty-nine hospitals into 'special measures' during the five years after it was introduced.[16] The impact on such hospitals was often profound: managers were dismissed, local newspapers devoted column inches to the issue and many staff felt upset. Given how hard they were working, that was sometimes unfair.

But it was still usually better than the alternative, which allowed poor care to persist as problems were concealed or swept under the carpet. That is because transparency forces large bureaucracies to act fast – and you need rapid change when patients' lives are at stake. None the less, the motive behind transparency matters too: rather than 'naming and shaming', it needs to focus on encouraging the sharing of best practice.

I remember meeting some NHS staff in a Manchester hospital that had recently gone into special measures. I was expecting a rough ride, but one of the staff unexpectedly put up his hand and instead of a question asked me to pass on a message to Bruce Keogh, then medical director of NHS England: 'Please tell him "thank you". Putting our hospital into special measures was painful. But in retrospect it was the best thing that ever happened to us. We needed something to push us into making change.'

9

Continuity

Dr Ronan Moran was perhaps the most down-to-earth doctor I ever met. The place I met him, though, was far from down to earth: at the glitz of a black-tie gala dinner at the Marriott in Grosvenor Square. The occasion was the *Daily Mail* Health Hero Awards.[1] I presented Dr Moran – the overall winner – with the top award that night. With characteristic humility he told me, 'I was just lucky to be the right person at the time. There are lots of doctors who are more worthy than I.'

Dr Moran ran a practice in Feltham, Middlesex that had been going for over thirty years. For much of that time he was the sole doctor there – what is known as a 'single-hander' practice. Such practices are not encouraged by the NHS, because they cannot offer a wide range of services. But Dr Moran liked it that way because he knew every patient and their families. They received what is known in medicine as 'continuity of care'.

One of those patients was James Walker, a former engineer who at seventy-six years old had been diagnosed with terminal cancer and discharged from hospital. Initially, his wife Grace felt rather abandoned at home after the hustle and bustle of the ward.

'After a few days, I realised that I wasn't on my own,' she said. 'Dr Moran was visiting, without being asked, and he was visiting every single day.'[2]

No hour was too late or inconvenient. During Mr Walker's last weeks in the autumn of 2011, Dr Moran visited him at home frequently, often late in the evening on his way home from work. He wouldn't let up even on weekends, particularly conscious that at such times his wife would end up dealing with a doctor new to James's case. If Mr Walker had had a bad night, Dr Moran would sit chatting with him about his favourite sport – Formula One – to try to lift his spirits.

When James passed away in the middle of one afternoon, Grace called the surgery. Dr Moran came round to certify the death. Once inside, he took off his jacket, rolled up his sleeves and began the quiet work of helping Mrs Walker wash her husband's body so that it would be ready to be taken away in a fresh set of clothes.

'I wanted him to leave his home with dignity,' he told me.

For many patients, having a family doctor is one of the most precious things about the NHS. The idea that there is someone who knows you and your family, indeed may have done for many years, is understandably popular with the public but also has significant clinical value. A study published in the *British Journal of General Practice* in 2021 showed that patients who have had the same GP for many years are 30% less likely to need hospital care, 30% less likely to use an out-of-hours service and 25% less likely to die.[3] Other important studies by Denis Pereira Gray and Richard Baker have suggested the same,[4] but this was the biggest study of its kind ever, using data from over four million Norwegian patients. It was widely welcomed by the UK's Royal College of GPs, because many doctors believe that building bonds over many years with the same families is more rewarding for doctors as well as better for patients.

But stories such as Ronan's have become increasingly rare.

Nearly two decades ago, the NHS scrapped the system that made GPs responsible for individual lists of patients. At the time, it was felt that it would be more efficient to attach patients to a surgery rather than an individual GP, meaning they saw the next available GP rather than their 'own' one. But even seeing one of a small group of GPs has become rarer: shortages of GPs have led to the widespread use of 'locum' or temporary doctors, meaning that the doctor you see at your surgery may be someone you never see again. Out-of-hours care has also become less personal: it used to be provided on a roster basis, organised by groups of surgeries in a locality. While you might not see your 'own' GP, you would at least be seen by someone from a neighbouring area. Now the care is provided under contract by organisations, often from the private sector, covering much larger areas.

As a result, for the first time in 2019 fewer than half of NHS patients said they had an ongoing relationship with a family doctor.[5] Many GPs, rushed off their feet, say it has now become utterly impossible to deliver such personalised care. We are rapidly moving to the Uberisation – where you are as unlikely to see the same GP as you are the same Uber driver – of general practice. The Norway study shows what a mistake this is, from the point of view not just of patient experience, but also patient usage of precious hospital beds. So is it too late to turn the clock back?

Before we consider that, I want to look at another story that illustrates that 'continuity of care', as it is called by professionals, is as important when it comes to hospital care as it is for general practice.

This was going to be a difficult meeting.

Jane Taylor had lost her husband Jeff after terrible failings in his care, and I was sitting next to her behind the large oval table in my office. Opposite us were three people I had invited to meet her – the chief executive, medical director and nursing director of the hospital where Jeff had been a patient.

Jane had sent me a long, handwritten letter detailing what had happened to Jeff. It had been 'selected' by the correspondence team for a personal reply by me, following my earlier request to start each day with a letter from a member of the public. The contents were very disturbing, so I decided to get to the bottom of what had happened.

That meeting was the first time Jane had come face to face with the people responsible for Jeff's care. She was visibly nervous. And so were they, not least because the meeting was being held in the Health Secretary's office. We started with Jane telling her story.

Jeff Taylor grew up in Stoke before becoming a heavy goods lorry driver. He met Jane in a pub in Barnsley and they got married in 1986. When he died, they had been married for nearly twenty-five years.

But Jeff was not just a regular lorry driver. He used to drive all over Europe and North Africa, often as part of aid missions. At the time of the Bosnian War, he worked for the UNHCR driving in supplies – mainly food and medicine – to Bosnia and Romania. In one incident, the driver who had taken his place was shot and killed by a sniper. On returning to the UK, Jeff battled PTSD for nearly a year.

His medical problems started when Jeff and Jane were on holiday in Lanzarote. While waiting at the airport, Jeff collapsed. He was taken to a nearby hospital. After an initial diagnosis, he was then airlifted to Gran Canaria. He had a blockage in his legs, so the doctors performed emergency surgery.

Jeff remained in hospital for six weeks. Eventually, he and Jane flew back to the UK on Boxing Day. But he still wasn't well. He had contracted a flesh-eating infection in the Spanish hospital that was eating into his groin. You could see right through his stomach where a bypass had been performed. He also had chronic diarrhoea, which had delayed their return home.

At first, Jane assumed that the diarrhoea was triggered by the amount of antibiotics he was on and that it would get better quickly. Nevertheless, it carried on so severely that she demanded further attention. She took Jeff to their local hospital where they saw a consultant, expecting immediate treatment.

Keen to make sure Jeff's medical history in Spain was known, Jane gave him a copy of the Spanish letter, detailing what had been done: two pages of notes about procedures, drugs and infections.

The consultant said that they would get it translated – which was absolutely vital, because without knowing how Jeff had been diagnosed and treated in Spain, it would be difficult to make sure he got the correct treatment now. Jane not only gave the consultant a physical copy of the letter, but also faxed a copy through to the nurse. She also made sure a copy was with the GP. Nothing was left to chance – but in the end not a word of that letter made its way onto Jeff's UK medical record.

In fact, according to Jane, the consultant was not remotely interested in what happened in Gran Canaria, apart from showing a certain 'we can do better than them' attitude. The consequences were dire.

After several weeks back in the UK, Jeff was still suffering from violent diarrhoea, sometimes twice an hour. He had lost a huge amount of weight, and was dangerously dehydrated.

But still the hospital wouldn't admit him. They sent him home and said he would get an emergency appointment with a vascular surgeon. It was the end of January before the emergency appointment materialised. But when they met the surgeon, he said he couldn't do anything until the diarrhoea was sorted out. So they had to book another appointment with a colorectal surgeon.

Jeff kept being pushed from pillar to post in different parts of the system. No single person was in charge. Never, at this stage, was he treated as an emergency patient.

As we sat there my mind was racing. I was horrified by the human misery that had unfolded – and the incompetence that lay behind it. But I also wanted to know if what Jane was telling us reflected the reality of the situation – was there another side to the story? But the senior team from the hospital made no attempt to question the facts being laid out. The chief executive seemed sympathetic, but the nursing director had a stony face.

Almost in response to some of the blank looks she was getting, Jane suddenly stopped mid-flow.

She brought out a photograph of her husband and passed it round the table. It was as if she wanted to remind us that Jeff was a real person. But the nursing director barely glanced at the picture. That same attitude had meant the hospital got Jeff's name wrong on every page in its documents.

The story continued with Jeff being given a stent in May, four months after his return from Lanzarote. The operation was scheduled for 7 May, but was cancelled and eventually performed on 20 May. They sat in the hospital for almost nine hours before they got a bed, because there was only one person cleaning the ward. The diarrhoea was at its worst, yet there was no help to be found.

After the stent was put in place, they were told to wait for six to eight weeks to see if things improved. In the meantime, they got a stairlift. They were told it was a six-month wait for a wheelchair.

Then, just as it seemed that progress was being made, the vascular surgeon literally disappeared. Jeff had gone into hospital for a follow-up appointment, but in an almost farcical scene the vascular surgeon left the room and never came back. Jane and Jeff didn't know it, but he had left the hospital.

It wasn't until July that they found out Jeff had a new vascular surgeon – but there was no handover whatsoever. It was back to square one.

The new vascular surgeon was the first person to look properly at Jeff's legs. By then he couldn't walk because of a 'dropped' foot. So the surgeon got Jeff seen by an orthopaedic consultant.

All it had needed was a brief ten-minute appointment to give Jeff a piece of plastic to put in his shoe to keep his foot up, which would have allowed him to start walking again. But by this time, serious damage had been done. Jeff hadn't been getting any physiotherapy, and by the time he had been home for a month without walking, his leg muscles had withered. None of which would have happened if that letter from the Spanish doctors had been translated.

Nor was the stent a success. After six weeks there was still no change, so the decision was made to schedule surgery for Jeff's bowel. Not optimal, but at least a solution, so he went to the hospital to have swabs and prepare for surgery. That night, however, he had a blocked artery in his leg, and had to be admitted as an emergency patient to have another bypass operation.

The bypass delayed Jeff's bowel surgery for yet another two months. Eventually, he got it done in November – *eleven months* after returning from Gran Canaria with chronic diarrhoea.

Jane hoped that at last things were finally being sorted. But worse was to come.

As they left the hospital following surgery, Jeff suddenly jerked with severe stomach pain. Jane told the doctor. But the doctor said it wasn't serious and they could go home.

The pain got worse, so a couple of days later Jane phoned for an ambulance. Jeff was always insistent that he didn't want to bother doctors and nurses, but Jane put her foot down.

Jeff was supposed to have immediate access to a surgical assessment unit, but that was refused. Left with no other option, she took him to A & E. In the meantime, the stoma bag Jeff had been given following the operation burst. In the rush to get the ambulance, Jane didn't have time to clean up. The stench was overwhelming.

On arrival at the hospital, Jeff remained in a state of trauma. Jane was told she could not clean Jeff up until a doctor had seen him. After more waiting, the doctor sent Jeff to the surgical assessment unit in a van. Despite having an agonising bowel condition, Jeff was propped up in a hard chair. When they put a seat belt round him, he cried out in pain.

On reaching the surgical assessment unit, it was another two-hour wait with just paracetamol to deaden the pain. Only then was Jane allowed to clean Jeff up. For six hours, waste had gone all over his dressings from the surgery and seeped into his wounds.

Jane began changing Jeff's bag, while the nurse changed his bandages for surgery. It was only then that the full horror of what had happened became apparent. When she came back, the nurse noticed that the waste wasn't coming from the bag. Jeff had faeces coming straight through his surgical scar. During the journey in the van and the wait for assessment, Jeff's bowel had burst.

He was immediately rushed to surgery. They were forced to take the rest of his bowel out, meaning that he could only survive with two stoma bags. He was in and out of theatre again over the coming days as complications arose, ending up with an irreparable hole in his stomach.

Jane went to see him in intensive care. It was when she was standing in the corridor, visitors and consultants passing by, that she was told the devastating truth.

Jeff was dying. She should warn the family.

But Jeff was stubborn.

Despite predictions that he might die within days, he lasted until Christmas. The problems continued: even though he had reacted badly to morphine in the past, Jeff was pumped full of it. He was then moved into a hospice and put on a course of intravenous feeding.

The end of the saga was as difficult as the beginning. Jeff was put on the end-of-life Liverpool Care Pathway, meaning that he was denied vital fluids. But in a major breach of protocol, Jane was not told.

From the moment Jeff collapsed in the queue at the airport, to over a year later when he died, it had been one long battle to get the care he deserved.

He never did.

Some of this had happened when I was Health Secretary. All of it had happened while my party was in power. There was no escaping responsibility, and I had a sinking feeling. A terrible tragedy had happened on my watch.

But *why* did things go so badly wrong?

It would be easy to dismiss the issue as 'bad apples' within the system – and the cold attitude of the nursing director did make me wonder whether that was the issue. Easy, too, to forget, when you hear Jeff's story, that other patients with similar conditions – the vast majority – would have been receiving outstanding care from the NHS at the same time. Even in the same hospital, I have no doubt there would have been excellent care being given to other patients.

But as we have seen from other stories, such incidents were far from unique. We have talked about the importance of transparency in ensuring that mistakes are properly aired and learned from. But here was a different issue: the lack of accountability for Jeff's care. Unlike what had happened with James Walker, there was no one in overall charge of his care. How else could it possibly have taken *eleven months* of appointments before Jeff's diarrhoea was sorted out?

The picture that emerges is of someone being pushed around the system by individuals who took responsibility – but only for their part of the process. The colorectal surgeon looked at the diarrhoea, the vascular specialist cared about issues relating to the veins, and so on – but no one took responsibility for the whole person, no one took charge of *Jeff*. Even though everyone was trying their best for their part of the process, collectively it was a shambles. Not once did anyone put themselves in Jeff's shoes and try to sort everything out.

Jeff's experience was not unique. Indeed, many patients with better connections and better resources than Jeff and Jane experience a similarly disjointed approach to their care. An Eton-educated fund manager who was at university with me told me about his recent diagnosis of prostate cancer. Having lived abroad under private insurance systems, he had become a massive fan of the NHS. But he could also be characterised as the ultimate 'patient with sharp elbows' – yet he, too, described a similarly disjointed approach to his care. On the positive side, thanks to the NHS, he had free access to some of the top specialists in the world. He benefited from 3D MRI scans that are not standard even in many other rich countries. He was also able to switch relatively easily from a generalist cancer centre to a world-renowned specialist hospital. His surgical care was superb.

But the lack of overall accountability for his care meant that he had to speak to six different members of the prostate team before he established which doctor would treat him. On each occasion, he had to repeat – as if on an assembly line – the details of his case and the treatment he thought he needed. When a tumour in his bladder was found to be benign, he was not told – because there was never a single point of contact to talk to. Letters and emails were never answered, and he felt that every time he needed treatment it was a fight to 'get back on the list', even though his was a fairly aggressive cancer. Some of this will have been exacerbated by the pandemic, but the lack of a single person responsible for his care long pre-dates Covid-19 – and was in essence the same problem that Jeff had faced.

Continuity of care matters. It allows a doctor to develop a contextual understanding of someone's family background, social situation and medical history – factors which can be essential for an accurate diagnosis. It gives patients security in a vulnerable situation. But it wasn't until I started coming across stories like Jeff's that I realised how dangerous the alternative can be, if patients are shifted between different doctors or teams without anyone taking overall responsibility.

However, my efforts to improve things had mixed results, to say the least.

I changed the GP contract to reintroduce the right to a 'named GP', first for patients over seventy-five years of age and then, in a later negotiation, for all patients.[6] Unfortunately, despite my high hopes, this turned into a 'tick-box' exercise, where patients often found no difference other than receiving a meaningless letter saying who their 'usual GP' was. I realised the main stumbling block was that we did not have enough GPs, which is why, in 2015, I announced the plan to increase the workforce by 5,000 over five years. As I mentioned earlier, an increase in those choosing to work part-time or retire early meant that the total headcount increased by only around three hundred over the following three years. Given how important it is to restore continuity of care, I hope that my successors do not give up on the task.

But improving numbers alone will not solve the issue.

In primary care, as well as returning to GPs having individual patient lists, the responsibility for a patient's care should be further strengthened by running district nurse and out-of-hours provision through groups of GP practices (possibly the new 'Primary Care Networks'), rather than regional NHS bureaucracies. That need not mean individual GPs having to be available 24/7 – but should mean they once again become accountable for ensuring good advice is given to their patients when a surgery is not open.

All changes should be based on moving back to the kind of care described in the Norway study, which has such a dramatic effect on both hospital attendance and mortality rates. In other words, they need to be real changes, not cosmetic ones, perhaps negotiated by replacing the current payment system (known as the Quality and Outcomes Framework) with higher year-round fees for each patient based on their age, health and social circumstances. Doing so would not only lead to less harm and greater longevity, but also end the toxic and distracting debate about whether people can see their GP face to face as opposed to virtually. Few people object to a phone or video consultation with a GP who actually knows them – and it can be more efficient for both parties. But if the doctor who sees you is someone who doesn't know you from Adam, the chance of an important clue being missed – say for a cancer – is much higher.

When it came to improving the accountability of hospital care, I reflected hard about cases like Jeff Taylor's. The then NHS England medical director, Bruce Keogh, worked with me to change NHS guidelines so that all hospitals were required to have a named consultant responsible for a patient's entire needs.[7] To make sure patients and families knew where the buck stopped, hospitals were encouraged to put boards above every bed with the name of the lead consultant and nurse written out clearly, something many hospitals have adopted. But, as with the attempts to introduce continuity of care in general practice, it has often ended up being little more than a tick-box exercise. One notable exception has been maternity care, where Chief Midwifery Officer Jacqueline Dunkley-Bent is ensuring that the majority of higher-risk pregnancies have the same team of midwives responsible for the care of mother and baby from the early stages, through the birthing process and in the post-natal period. To deliver this consistently will, however, require more midwives than we currently have.

But whether inside or outside hospital, we need a decisive change in the model of care offered by the NHS, so that patients *always* have one doctor or nurse clearly responsible for their care. In normal circumstances that should be a patient's GP, although for frail elderly patients it might be a district nurse. But if a patient with complex needs, like Jeff, has to go to hospital, they should be kept under the supervision of a single consultant even when elements of their care are performed by other specialists. Then, when a patient is discharged, responsibility should be transferred carefully back to their GP.

We need to do this not just to avoid extreme cases when things go wrong, but because patients like Jeff are becoming more common. Life expectancy is now around eighty-one years in both the UK and the US,[8] but a more meaningful figure is what is called 'healthy life expectancy' – the number of years we can expect to live free of major ailments. This is rather lower, seventy-two years in the UK and sixty-nine years in the US.[9] What that means is that many people can expect about a decade of poor health at the end of their lives, when they have to battle multiple chronic conditions. This makes it more likely that they will need complex help during a hospital visit – for which clear lines of accountability are essential.

The issue of accountability for care – and its importance in reducing avoidable harm and death – extends beyond the NHS. Local authorities are responsible for social care in England, and too often patients are pushed from pillar to post as arguments rage between the health and care systems about who should take budgetary responsibility for someone's treatment. I came across a powerful example of this in my current role as chair of the Health and Social Care Select Committee, when we took evidence during the pandemic from a member of the public called Daphne Havercroft.[10] She talked about the extreme distress caused to her 96-year-old mother Dorothy Boschi, who spent fourteen months at the end of her life being ferried between random hospital and care home beds.

Dorothy was living at home, with support from her family who lived nearby. She ended up needing to go to hospital three times – and never returned home after the second admission. Instead, she spent seven months in hospital and six months in a temporary residential care placement. A palliative care package that would have allowed her to go home was requested by doctors but never provided; no explanation was ever given, but her family assumes it was because neither the NHS nor her local authority were prepared to fund it. She ended up dying in a nursing home fourteen months after her initial admission.

Her family believe that all three of her emergency admissions could have been avoided if she had been given better support at home, with a single plan put in place to anticipate and deal with the symptoms of her vascular dementia. While her hospital care was excellent insofar as it went, as with Jeff Taylor, it was not part of any larger plan to look after her. Because there was no integrated working between health and care professionals, Dorothy was put under enormous stress, causing her dementia to deteriorate much more quickly.

Even putting such suffering aside, what Dorothy went through made no financial sense. A hospital bed costs at least £300 a night,[11] but a bed in a care home £100 a night[12] and a homecare package typically £50, depending on hours worked.[13] Sorting out Dorothy's care so she could spend that last year at home or in a care home would have cost both the NHS and care system less. She ended up being looked after by a total of 101 different professionals – including both those who met her and provided care, and those who worked on her case behind the scenes – at enormous expense. Far more cost-effective, as her daughter Daphne points out, would have been to look after her better at home so that she would not need to go to hospital in the first place.

Of course, such funding needs to be provided 'up front' – and can take several years to feed through into reduced hospital budgets. It

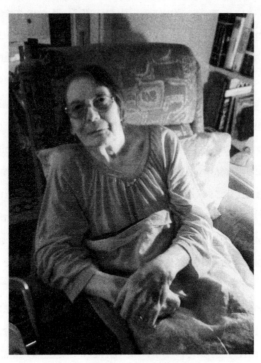

Dorothy Boschi

therefore requires a superhuman effort for policymakers to find the resources for such measures, in other words to switch the focus to preventing ill health rather than putting it right. But it is easier than it was: the kind of remote care that would help someone like Dorothy is now becoming much more affordable thanks to advances in technology. The University of Surrey, for example, has developed a remote monitoring system that detects if someone has a fall.[14] It can even monitor if someone doesn't put the kettle on in the morning to make a cup of tea. If that sounds intrusive, remember that for Dorothy such a system might have meant she could stay in her own home indefinitely rather than move to a care home. That might have made it a decision that she and her family would have been happy to make.

Given that, in the UK, hospital costs – and often care home costs – are funded by taxpayers, you might think that the UK would have twigged earlier the financial sense of adopting such an approach. As an American health insurer once told a colleague of mine:

> In the US, we are taught that if you acquire a customer for one year you lose money, as their claims will cost more than their premium. Hold on to them for three years, and with good care you can keep their costs below what they pay in premiums. But if you get them for seven years, you can really teach them how to stay healthy, and that's when you make money. In the NHS you have customers for their whole life – so you should be making a fortune, right?

When most costs are borne by the state, as in the UK, the incentive to invest in low-cost prevention of illness rather than higher-cost treatment is much greater than in private systems such as the US, where the extra cost falls back on individuals. But the setting up of an internal market, followed by the Lansley reforms, meant the NHS ignored this logic. A 'payment by results' system – known as 'fee for service' in the US – means NHS hospitals have long been incentivised to maximise the number of operations they perform.[15] On top of this, underfunding of the social care system has prevented close collaboration with the NHS, because it is wary of taking on additional financial liabilities. The result is that instead of sitting down and working out what would be in Dorothy's best interest – which would also have kept her out of hospitals and care homes and therefore been much cheaper too – arguments over demarcation and budgetary responsibility mean the patient comes last.

If we really want to stop stories like Dorothy's being repeated, we should merge the health and care systems. That is a big job. But we could start more modestly within the current systems, by making sure vulnerable people have a single, agreed care plan and a single person responsible for every patient. All details need to be accessible electronically by professionals in either system through a single health and care record, an idea we will return to later.

None of those reforms will happen without a long-term plan for the social care system. It needs to sit alongside – and be consistent with – the ten-year plan we now have for the NHS. Such a plan needs to ensure not only that people like Dorothy are treated in a consistent, compassionate way, but also to deal with some obvious issues, such as the funding available for local authorities, the unfairness of the catastrophic care costs faced by a small minority of families dealing with dementia or other neurological conditions, and an utterly demoralised workforce, where low pay and a career structure with much less opportunity for advancement than in the NHS means that annual staff turnover is around a third. How can good care be delivered by any organisation if they are losing a third of their workforce every year?

Germany and Japan have both addressed these issues successfully.[16] Both have a social insurance and risk pooling system in which older people pay more in taxes in return for more security around their care in old age. In Germany, the support you receive can even be used to pay family members, which is very different to the approach taken in the UK. Unusually, given the unpopularity of tax rises, in both Germany and Japan the social consensus supports the bold approach their governments have taken. Although our government has made some first, halting steps in the right direction, we do not yet have a plan of similar imagination and ambition.

However, reform is now finally starting to happen, albeit slowly.

In Farnham, in my own constituency, the local hospital, Frimley Park, has joined up with GPs and community providers to form the Frimley Health and Care Integrated Care System. Teams of nurses look after vulnerable older people in their homes, with referrals coming directly from any local GP concerned about a patient. A & E consultants refer patients directly to that team, allowing them to be sent home sooner without having to be admitted to hospital. By the third year of the scheme, pretty much for the first time anywhere in the country, emergency admissions started falling at the hospital. Patients, too, are noticing the difference, as I can see from my MP postbag. Similar models are being tried successfully in South Yorkshire and Bassetlaw, Suffolk and North East Essex and Dorset. When it comes to joining up the health and care systems, change has been slower, but around one in ten local authorities have started to merge the two systems.

Unless such changes happen faster and in more places, stories like those of Jeff Taylor and Dorothy Boschi will continue to jolt and shock.

10

Homecare

Connor Sparrowhawk was born with autism and epilepsy. He was an extremely happy boy – indeed, his nickname was Laughing Boy. His family and friends loved him, and he loved them back. Then, in his last year at secondary school, he started to show aggressive traits. No one really knew why, although many young people with autism struggle hard with adolescence. Perhaps it was the prospect of his friends going to university without him that brought home the limitations he faced. At any rate, he ended up being admitted to a small NHS unit near Oxford as a voluntary patient.

However, within four hours he was restrained face down on the floor and then sectioned under the Mental Health Act. His mother Sara Ryan was so concerned about the care he was receiving that she documented her concerns in a blog.[1] Her fears crystallised a few months later, when he had an epileptic seizure while having a bath. He should have been supervised, but no one had considered the risk of allowing him to bathe alone. At the age of eighteen, he drowned.

We have heard about many such tragedies so far, and in this section we will be looking at the key solutions. Better continuity of care, as discussed in the last chapter, would have made a big difference to

Connor's welfare. But we will now focus on another issue specific to the needs of autistic people and those with learning disabilities: the importance of appropriate care at home or in community settings, as opposed to being 'parked' for long periods of time – even indefinitely – in locked units, which can make their condition even worse. Alongside people with severe mental illness, these two groups of people often find it hardest to get their voices heard, which means they have a much greater chance of experiencing preventable harm, something we will see from what happened when Connor's mother tried to get to the bottom of his death.[2]

The NHS trust responsible for Connor's care is called Southern Health, and its chief executive was an NHS high-flyer called Katrina Percy. She had a formidable reputation, having overseen the successful merger of the Hampshire community and mental health services, and then a subsequent merger with services in Oxfordshire and Buckinghamshire. She had earned the coveted accolade of *Health Service Journal* Chief Executive of the Year.[3]

When Connor died, she was away on maternity leave but his death was discussed at a board meeting. After that meeting, the minutes recorded that Connor's death was from 'natural causes'. Sara was furious – it just seemed to confirm her worst fears of a cover-up. The trust appeared to be following an all too standard playbook: concede nothing and fight off the 'troublesome' relatives. As we will see, the trust had a different explanation for what happened, which Katrina Percy explained to me when we met. But for Sara, insult was added to injury when she discovered that a rebuttal email was sent round addressing some of the claims she had made in her blog.

Her relationship with the trust then broke down.

Not unreasonably, Sara insisted that any investigation into Connor's death had to be independent. She requested to see Connor's medical notes, from which her solicitor identified numerous areas of concern. Finally – despite heavy resistance from the trust – she persuaded a coroner to do what is called an 'Article 2 inquest', used when there is the possibility of a wrongful death in the care of the state.

She also tweeted at David Nicholson, then chief executive of the NHS, requesting a meeting. To his credit he agreed to this immediately, and when she went to see him accepted her request for an independent review into all the unexpected deaths that had happened at the trust. The report became mired in controversy over its methodology inside the NHS, which meant that its publication kept on being delayed. It was eventually leaked to a journalist and its findings were explosive: of 337 unexpected deaths of patients with a learning disability since the trust was formed, only two had been investigated.[4] I was the Health Secretary, and was summoned to parliament to answer questions about it.

The trust fought back, saying that they were not the primary care-giver for many of the 337 unexpected deaths. Sara took her family to a public board meeting, at which Connor's brother Tom, just sixteen years old, challenged Katrina Percy as to why she had not met with the family to apologise face to face for what had happened. Katrina Percy says the offer of meeting had previously been made but not accepted – but she made a split-second decision not to say that to a sixteen-year-old boy. Ultimately she ended up resigning from the trust.

Meanwhile, Sara enlisted the support of Norman Lamb, who worked for me as a minister and was the staunchest and most impressive advocate of mental health and learning disability issues I had ever come across. With Norman's help, Sara persuaded the HSE to reopen an investigation into the deaths of Connor and another patient called Teresa Colvin, who had died two years earlier. In November 2017, the trust pleaded guilty to corporate manslaughter and the following March was given a £2 million fine, the biggest such fine in the history of the NHS at the time.[5] The judge paid tribute to Sara's extraordinary campaigning and said that if the trust had learned properly from Teresa's death Connor might still be alive.

In researching this book, I decided to meet not just Sara Ryan but also Katrina Percy.

I wasn't sure if either would be willing to meet, but in fact both were happy to discuss what happened and what lessons could be learned. Their accounts of what happened do not differ in the most important respect: both think Connor's death could and should have been avoided. Katrina Percy accepts she should have handled things differently. But she also explained how challenging it was for her as a CEO to cope with the situation, including the intense media scrutiny of her personally at the same time as running a large organisation.

The relationship between Sara and the trust broke down irretrievably – and passed the point of no return at the board meeting when Connor's death was recorded as resulting from 'natural causes'. But what had really happened at that meeting was a board discussion about whether the death was the result of suicide or foul play. The police had concluded it was neither, so the phrase 'natural causes' was used by the board secretary. It wasn't meant to suggest that the death was not preventable, but understandably was interpreted as such by Sara. Had there been better communication between the NHS and the bereaved family, that misunderstanding might not have arisen.

The critical mistake in Connor's care seems to have been a failure to assess the risks arising from his epilepsy. That possibly happened because, in a perverse piece of bureaucracy, his epilepsy – but not his other health issues – was being managed by a different NHS organisation, the John Radcliffe in Oxford. A properly shared electronic health record might have helped – but nursing basics would also have suggested that it was an inappropriate risk to allow him to bathe alone.

Given his disability, a special effort should have been made with his care – but was not.

Those errors were then compounded by multiple failures in the way Southern Health responded to the tragedy.

What needed to happen was a rapid, thorough investigation of the processes that led to Connor's death, alongside improvements to make sure it could not happen again. Instead, the focus switched overwhelmingly to the performance of Katrina Percy, even though she had been away on maternity leave when the tragedy happened.

No organisation can prevent staff members making mistakes from time to time, but it can at least make sure any tragedy is responded to appropriately. In this case, corporate mergers may have led to the trust board being distracted. The board members faced big organisational challenges when they were asked to take on Oxfordshire's and Buckinghamshire's troubled learning disability services just a few months before Connor's death. Those challenges became even more acute when the clinical director responsible for learning disability services resigned, rather leaving them in the lurch. Did such events contribute to poor oversight of the care of Connor and others? It is impossible to know. But it is clear this was not a board that could give its undiluted attention to the quality of care it delivered.

What about my role, sitting on top of the pyramid? Did I handle the conflict between Sara Ryan and Katrina Percy as well as I could have? Probably not.

As Health Secretary, you are several layers away from what is happening. But ultimately you are responsible for everything that happens on your watch including, in this case, Connor's death. You can never prevent every error, but I wish I had intervened earlier to get Sara the answers she sought about Connor's care.

I also wish our focus had moved more quickly to putting right the system's failures, rather than the mistakes made by an otherwise exemplary NHS chief executive. Katrina Percy ended up becoming the flashpoint for all that went wrong with Connor's care, and has paid a high personal price. She now uses a different last name, is unable to work in the NHS and has suffered enormous mental stress. She describes extensive social media trolling, aggressive media intrusion and neighbours looking at her as if she was a murderer.

Of course, NHS leaders – and the politicians they report to – should be accountable for any mistakes on their watch. But sometimes what I would describe as 'rotten apple syndrome' means large organisations find it easier to deal with problems by focusing on an individual rather than system failures. Is it fair or wise to write off someone as a rotten apple based on one badly handled case, however serious? The risk in doing so is that despite apparent 'accountability', system failures that may have been the primary cause of a tragedy remain uncorrected.

Those system failings are still far from being addressed – and while there are many broader lessons to be learned from this story, it also illustrates the particular vulnerability of people with learning disabilities. They have a life expectancy at least fourteen years shorter for men and eighteen years shorter for women. They were up to six times more likely to die in the Covid-19 pandemic.[6] Sara talks about a culture around autism and learning disability in which patient harm and death is treated as 'collateral damage'. She talks about the 'infallibility myth' surrounding doctors that makes it hard to admit mistakes. She describes receiving the same abuse for asking questions about Connor's care that Julie Bailey and Deb Hazeldine received after Mid Staffs.

And stories like Connor's are part of a bigger pattern.

Similar issues were identified in a report into the care of a 56-year-old woman with learning disabilities called Annette, over a four-year period in South Yorkshire. She was forcibly restrained without justification, given the wrong doses of medication and not protected from other violent patients. She was finally diagnosed with cancer – just two days before she died from it in 2014, starkly illustrating the link between her learning disability and cancer care that is vastly inferior to what most people would receive.

Rotherham, Doncaster and South Humber Trust did eventually commission an independent report into her care which catalogued these failings. It identified a failure to listen to Annette's family as being a key issue. In both Annette's and Connor's cases, families played an essential role in giving a voice to people who find it difficult to express their own feelings and emotions. The trust apologised 'in full and without reservation'.[7]

Dealing openly with tragedies such as those of Connor and Annette so that lessons can be learned is only, however, the tip of the iceberg when it comes to preventing avoidable harm to the most vulnerable groups. Poor care has also become part of the structure. In Britain today, we still forcibly detain large numbers of people with autism, learning disabilities or severe mental illnesses in what are known as 'assessment and treatment units' or 'locked rehab' facilities, instead of supporting them to live in the community, which they would be perfectly capable of doing.[8]

Often, the problem starts when individuals or their families seek help during a crisis and agree that someone can become an inpatient in 'secure' accommodation on a supposedly temporary basis. Such units are often run by private or independent sector providers charging thousands of pounds a week. But 'temporary' turns out to be quite the opposite – the average length of stay is currently more than five and a half years, stretching up to a decade for around one in ten patients.

Part of the reason they get 'stuck' in locked rehab is that their bills are picked up by the NHS, not the cash-strapped local authorities who might otherwise pay for support in the community. Local authorities are quite happy to leave such patients somewhere where funding is not their responsibility – and in fairness often lack the resources to do any differently. But the result of such institutional buck-passing is that over 2,000 people are currently incarcerated in such units in England, even though the CQC says many could live independently in the community.[9]

In some such facilities, terrible abuse can occur – as in the infamous case of Winterbourne View hospital in Gloucestershire. This was exposed by a BBC *Panorama* programme in 2011, which detailed evidence of residents being assaulted by staff, restrained harshly and given cold showers or left outside in freezing temperatures as punishment. One patient tried to jump out of a window to escape and was mocked by staff for doing so.[10]

Despite repeated requests, both the NHS and the CQC did not address the issue – but the *Panorama* programme finally forced a change of heart. David Cameron, the Prime Minister at the time, said publicly that he was appalled, and ultimately eleven members of staff were convicted of multiple charges of neglect and ill treatment, with six going to jail.[11] The hospital was closed, alongside three more run by Castlebeck Care, which was responsible for it.[12] Yet a string of other recent exposés by broadcasters and newspapers, backed by damning official inquiries, have shown that such abuse was far from unique, including a recent one at Yew Trees private hospital in Essex, run by Cygnet Health.[13] All too often, citizens seeking support end up being held in conditions that are simply inhumane, intensifying any mental health problems and tearing families apart. One teenage girl with autism was held in solitary confinement and fed through a hatch on the floor, with the local council taking her father to court when he sought publicity to help his child.[14]

Even in units where there is no outright abuse (and no *Panorama* programme to expose it), residents are often subjected to forced medication or the use of 'restraint' – physical force to control challenging behaviour. The use of restraint can be extremely traumatic, but is generally completely unnecessary, when someone moves out of an institutional environment into the community. Even inside an institution, proper training in understanding the needs of individuals with autism or learning disabilities can reduce or even eliminate the use of such practices – tension is reduced by more cooperative and less stressful relationships. But all too often the effect of an institutional environment is the dehumanisation of both residents and staff.

So why not close them down?

In 1978, Italy took the radical step of banning all such asylums – for that is what they really are.[15] It passed a law to prohibit long-stay mental health units half a century ago, inspired by the work of a radical psychiatrist called Franco Basaglia who became famous for freeing 1,200 patients from a huge asylum in Trieste. Asylums were replaced with general hospitals and community-led provision. The campaigning journalist Ian Birrell told me that one telling side effect of this reform in Trieste was that some formerly abusive staff, forced to treat their charges as human beings rather than inmates, ended up caring for the same people with great sensitivity.

Some progress has been made in the UK. Norman Lamb and I made efforts to transfer as many people with learning disabilities into the community as we could, under the 'Transforming Care' programme. We found it to be an immensely complicated process, as the needs of each individual were so different – and sadly many had become institutionalised over the years. But too often the problem was an underdeveloped support infrastructure in the communities where they should have been living. Even though that can be expensive, it is usually much cheaper than keeping them in an institution – as well as being vastly more humane.

We should follow Italy's example and close all the 'locked rehab' and 'assessment and treatment units', banning the long-term admission of new patients with autism, learning disabilities and mental health conditions except when people have committed crimes. We closed our mental health asylums in the 1980s and 1990s with an extremely successful programme that transferred people into supported living in the community.[16] But when it came to people with autism and learning disabilities, we never finished the job. Until we do, we risk a repeat of what happened at Winterbourne View.

There may well be a need for patients to stay temporarily in secure assessment centres, but if so, we should do as they do in Italy, where the authorities have to reapply to 'section' patients every week, rather than every six months as in England. We should also recognise that many organisations that look after people with challenging conditions on a long-term basis do so with the very highest standards of care and compassion, such as the Meath in Godalming, in my own constituency. Any solution must leave room for such beacons of humanity.

More broadly, these issues – whether in individual cases such as Connor's or Annette's, or as a result of large-scale structural inhumanity such as the supposedly 'temporary' 'assessment and treatment units' – illustrate the particular danger faced by people not able to advocate for themselves. Because out of sight can so easily be out of mind, any reform programme to reduce avoidable harm and death needs to take special care to address such risks.

Thanks to campaigning by Sara Ryan and others, a number of positive changes have finally happened. The NHS responded to what happened to Connor with a national programme designed to make sure all unexpected deaths are properly investigated. It finally put in place the Medical Examiners programme which means that every hospital death is now checked by a second, independent doctor.[17] The law was also changed to require all hospitals to publish their own estimate of the number of avoidable deaths of patients in their care, although that has not yet been properly implemented.

There have also been other improvements: following campaigning by Paula McGowan after the untimely death of her son Oliver in 2016, mandatory training in learning disabilities for health and care staff was introduced in 2019, known as Oliver McGowan Mandatory Training, 'in recognition of Oliver's story, his family's tireless campaigning for better training for staff, and to remember him and others whose lives were cut tragically short'.[18] This should help address one of the biggest issues, which is a failure to diagnose physical health problems in a group of people often unable to express themselves. To tackle the over-medication of people with learning disabilities with anti-psychotic drugs, a programme called STOMP is underway.[19] But given how little we still understand the complex interaction between learning disabilities and a range of other conditions, there should probably be a new medical specialty that focuses on learning disability, as well as a requirement for GPs to offer regular physical health checks to people who may not come forward in the same way other patients do.

But even after such changes have been made, the scale of the overall injustice facing people with autism and learning disabilities remains shocking. Two thousand people remain under lock and key, the majority of whom could be living happily and independently in the community. A disturbing number of avoidable fatalities are still happening within the health system. Mencap's analysis of the 2021 annual report on the deaths of people with learning disabilities (known as the LeDeR programme) found that 'people with a learning disability died from an avoidable medical cause of death twice as frequently as people in the general population'.[20] Until we transform the community care available for some of our most vulnerable citizens, that picture will not change.

11

Prevention

Melissa Mead has become the country's most formidable sepsis campaigner. She started as an ordinary mum from Cornwall – but then tragedy struck when she lost her one-year-old son William.

When we met she was clutching William's teddy bear. She placed it on the table in front of her as she told her story. I assumed it was to remind us about the child at the centre of the tragedy. Only afterwards did I find out that inside that teddy were William's ashes.

She took those ashes with her not just to her meeting with me, but to every meeting she went to in her quest to find out the truth about his death. She took it to every newspaper interview. She took it into every TV studio. The impact she had was enormous and her work on sepsis prevention has saved many lives.

During that first encounter, I could sense both anger and suspicion in her eyes. She had come on a long and painful journey. Was she about to be fobbed off by yet another politician who failed to match words with action?

In September 2014, William was a healthy child coming up to his first birthday. He had just started nursery. One day he came back with a heavy cold. After going to the doctor's he was diagnosed with acute tonsillitis and prescribed antibiotics.

The symptoms didn't go away, but Melissa was advised it was just a winter cold. This seemed to make sense as he had just started going to nursery, often thought to be 'super-spreader' environments. 'Don't worry,' the GP told Melissa with a knowing smile, 'remember you are a first-time mum.'

But she had to go back to that same doctor a few weeks later because William started coughing up mucus and vomiting. He was also losing weight. The doctor decided the loss of baby fat was down to his having started to move around a lot as he got ready to walk. On 27 November, still not better, he celebrated his first birthday.

Then, on a Friday in mid-December, his nursery called Melissa to say they were putting him to bed because he was not well. She took him to the GP that evening, but at the end of a busy week he was only given a cursory examination. The GP identified his temperature was 40.1 degrees, but said it was a virus. In fact, it was a bacterial infection that was already turning into sepsis. One of his lungs had already collapsed.

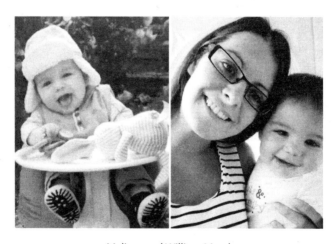

Melissa and William Mead

Melissa and her partner Paul were planning to leave for Spain the next week to join Melissa's parents for Christmas. Without telling Melissa, Paul had secretly booked a registry office wedding for them on the Monday morning ahead of the trip. It was going to be a Christmas of surprises and celebration.

But William was still unwell.

His temperature started coming down on the Saturday morning, but because he was so weak Melissa decided to call the 111 helpline. The call handler, who was not clinically trained, followed a computer-generated algorithm that told him what questions to ask. However, he mis-entered some of Melissa's answers, so the algorithm booked her in for a 'six-hour callback' by a doctor instead of an emergency ambulance. When the callback eventually happened, the doctor was reading the answers mis-entered by the call handler. Melissa didn't know this, and was told William would be 'right as rain' in the morning. So she cuddled him goodnight and told him she loved him.

They were her last ever words to her son. When she went in to see him at half past eight the next morning, he was dead.

As I listened, I couldn't stop myself doing some sums in my head. William, I realised, was just eight months older than my youngest daughter. Everything that happened to him could have happened to her. *That could have been us.* The thought was terrifying.

Even though it was too late, Melissa explained that from that point on the system moved very fast. Paramedics arrived in just three minutes and forty-four seconds. Frantically, they tried CPR for seven minutes. 'I'm sorry, love, but he's gone,' they told Melissa. Still in her pyjamas, she climbed in the back of the ambulance that took William's body to the hospital.

When she got home the next day, she lay on the floor in William's bedroom and cried – on the very day she was supposed to be getting married.

Melissa's campaigning since then has helped transform our under-standing of sepsis. But the defensive culture we saw at Joshua Titcombe's and Elaine Bromiley's hospitals was just as strong in the community environment responsible for William's care. Melissa found it impossible to get anyone to admit anything had gone wrong.

The GP surgery did a 'serious event audit'. But Melissa was not involved in it at all, and the conclusion came back that 'nothing could have been done differently'.

Only when the coroner said there would be an inquest did Melissa realise something might have gone wrong. Melissa and Paul asked the coroner why their concerns were repeatedly ignored. They questioned why no tests were conducted – no chest X-rays, no blood tests, no saliva samples – on that final Friday when William was taken in. They wanted to know why the doctor did not spot William's collapsed lung.

Unfortunately, the result of the inquest was no more satisfactory. Child death inquests are only done once a month in Cornwall, and coroners generally aim to get through three in a day. Because of Melissa's questions, William's inquest took a whole day. But towards the end of the proceedings Melissa noticed the coroner producing a pre-written typed-up verdict, suggesting she had already made up her mind before hearing the evidence. That seemed to be confirmed by the verdict – 'death by natural causes'.

However, Melissa did not give up.

She enrolled the support of her local MP, Sarah Newton. After more than six hundred emails, Melissa eventually persuaded the NHS to do a 'root cause analysis' that brought together all the agencies involved in William's care. Melissa then badgered the NHS to make sure the review was truly independent.[1]

At the start, the signs were not encouraging: 'Melissa, dear, these things happen,' she was told by one of the people conducting the review.

In the end, though, the final report was accurate. It found no fewer than sixteen failings in William's care, including four missed chances to save his life. A far cry from 'nothing could have been done differently'.

One of those missed chances was the 111 call, made on the day before William died. The call – in a rather over-scientific way – was assessed as being only '76% compliant' with the standards required (against a minimum required level of 86% compliance). A whistle-blower contacted Melissa secretly to tell her that the original internal analysis had shown the call was only 47% compliant – and had then been doctored to make the breach look less serious.

She was experiencing exactly the same defensiveness and blame culture that James Titcombe had with the Morecambe Bay midwives who 'lost' Joshua Titcombe's medical records. People were afraid to be open, perhaps because they thought they would lose their jobs, perhaps because they had persuaded themselves things happened differently to how they actually did, the 'memory illusion'. The fact that in each case the stories were splashed on the front pages of local newspapers will also have raised the tension in the situation.

But as we have seen with so many stories in this book, the only way to learn lessons is to confront the truth, however uncomfortable. And in this case Melissa's GP did finally apologise. 'He is a good doctor who will never make that mistake again. And next time he will save a child's life,' she now says graciously. 'The best apology is changed behaviour.'

According to the WHO, the sepsis that killed William is one of the biggest causes of preventable death worldwide.[2] It is also totally treatable – if caught early. Prevention is better than cure – and one of the key solutions to reducing the levels of avoidable harm and death. Having explored the importance of transparency and continuity of care, in this chapter we will look at how much patient harm could be prevented from arising in the first place.

In William's case, that would have meant both clinicians and the public understanding more clearly the risk of sepsis. Thanks to brilliant campaigning by Melissa and a small charity called the UK Sepsis Trust,[3] this has now started to happen, with public awareness of the disease improving markedly. Ambulances now have 'Could it be sepsis?' posters on their sides and thousands of leaflets have been distributed to GP surgeries. In a relatively short time clinical practice has also changed significantly, with big rises in the number of patients screened for sepsis when they arrive in an A & E.[4] The 'Sepsis Six' care bundle is used in nine out of ten hospitals. But the most important change for Melissa is the way doctors and nurses are now encouraged to listen to parents who say something is not right. Parents know their children best, and even doctors with the best training need to tap into the instincts of parents if a hidden killer is to be tackled.

I apologised publicly for the failings in William's care at a memorial service in Truro Cathedral, a gesture that was met with great generosity by his family. But despite the success of their campaigning, Melissa paid an enormous personal price. Carrying William's ashes around TV studios boosted sepsis awareness – but it made it harder for her personally to move on, leading at one point to an attempt to take her own life. The last time I spoke to her, she was moving house. She told me the biggest wrench was saying goodbye to William's bedroom. Like many bereaved parents, she had turned it into a shrine to remember him by. 'The only thing William wanted was life,' she said, 'and I am not going to waste mine.' She has not – as shown by the many lives she has saved through her sepsis campaigning.

'Prevention' has become something of a buzzword in medicine. At its broadest, it covers public health issues like smoking and obesity. Tackling such issues is vitally important, although beyond the scope of this book. But prevention is important in any clinical process too: if the people caring for William had spotted his sepsis earlier, he would still be alive. Knowledge of potential diseases matters – as does knowing the risks in medication administration. Here, too, better training and more robust systems can make a big difference in preventing avoidable harm and death.

The NHS dispenses roughly six million prescriptions every day, of which getting on for half are not in hospitals but in the community.[5] Sometimes tragedies happen because of unscrupulous behaviour by drugs companies: the use of Distaval resulted in many children being born with deformities in the 1950s and 1960s, a tragedy that became known as the thalidomide scandal.[6] In that case, the drug manufacturer continued to distribute Distaval despite being aware of the risks. As Health Secretary, I dealt with several issues with disturbing similarities, including the use of sodium valproate, an epilepsy drug that, if taken during pregnancy, sometimes caused children to be born with a disability. A very experienced and competent former health minister, Julia Cumberlege, conducted a thorough review of what went wrong.[7]

But often, harm caused by medication error is much less high profile, caused not by profiteering drugs companies but by the inevitable human error that happens with so many prescriptions and so much dispensing. Such errors may have contributed to Jack Adcock's death, which I described earlier. After hearing a few similar stories, I decided to gather a group of patients together in my office to try to understand the issue better.

One man described how his 84-year-old mother was poisoned after being given the wrong dose of lithium. She wasn't monitored and, in the end, died an excruciatingly painful death, having to be strapped to her bed to keep her still. Another woman described how her 92-year-old mother, with vascular dementia, had her medical records muddled up with those of someone else who had the same name. The pharmacist didn't notice, the care home didn't notice – in the end it was her own daughter who did. She survived a further three and a half years before dying in terrible pain.

The most harrowing story concerned a redoubtable lady called Fiona Hogan, who was a retired probation officer from Blackpool. Her job involved doing risk assessments within the court system – including the enormous responsibility of signing off whether high-risk offenders such as murderers and sex-offenders were safe to be let back into the community. She combined this with a happy family life, including – now – four grandchildren.

Two weeks before one Christmas, the vision in her left eye started getting blurred, so she went to the Blackpool Victoria Hospital. She was admitted for three days and prescribed 50 mg of steroids to be taken daily, after which she was referred to the Royal Liverpool's St Paul's Eye Unit for an appointment after Christmas.

There she was told they wanted to 'zap it again', so was again given 50 mg of steroids for three days. Because of the strength of the medicine – she was on the highest dose allowed – she was told it could only be at that level for three days. Her GP was given instructions to reduce the dose to 7.5 mg after the weekend. To double-check her GP got the instructions, Fiona was given a piece of paper to hand over to him.

Subsequently, all her records stated her dosage had been reduced to 7.5 mg daily – but in fact the change was not made. Fiona continued on the much higher dosage, 50 mg a day, unnoticed by any of the doctors or pharmacists looking after her.

She started to develop strange symptoms. She began to find it difficult to eat, started losing weight and her joints started aching. Because she was still having monthly appointments, she was referred for tests. Her doctors became convinced it was an autoimmune condition. Her tests revealed she was developing ulcers from her throat right the way through to her stomach, but no one could understand why. Because her records still said she was on 7.5 mg, no one thought it was the steroids. Nor did anyone check the dosage.

This carried on not just for a few weeks or months, but for a shocking *six years*. Then, finally, an investigation revealed the cause as being the high dosage of steroids being put on a repeat prescription. By then it was too late. To have such a high dose even for a month would make someone steroid-dependent. Her body was wrecked. She cannot now eat through her mouth at all, and gets her nutrition through a tube in her stomach. She describes swallowing cold water as being as painful as putting glass down your throat. Her body still craves steroids.

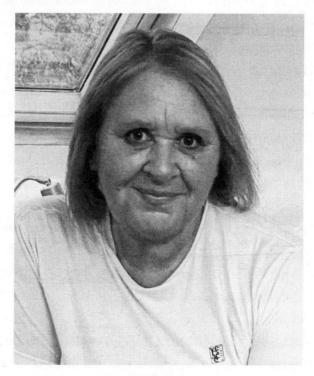

Fiona Hogan

The GP who, according to Fiona, had failed to change her dosage had retired by then. He happens to live near Fiona, but has never spoken to her since. She was, however, given a fulsome apology by the local surgery, who said its systems had subsequently changed. But as Fiona explains, this was a far cry from what would have happened in the probation world where she had made her career. If a mistake was made when an offender was released, there was a full inquiry, with all notes examined by someone independent. Instead, it was explained to Fiona that, with millions of prescriptions issued every year, some error was 'inevitable'. To her credit, she has remained a totally positive person throughout, cheerfully telling me how her grandchildren now describe her: 'Granny can't eat, but she can drink gin.'

Prompted by such stories, in 2017 I commissioned the universities of Sheffield, Manchester and Leeds to put together a report reviewing all the academic studies on medication error. I asked them to quantify the extent of the harm caused in the NHS. The results that came back showed Fiona's experience was just the tip of the iceberg.

The researchers said there were 66 million 'clinically significant' medication errors every year – or over one million a week. Compared to the 5 million people treated by the NHS every week, that is a large number. Most such errors will have had no long-term effect, but the research estimated that adverse drug reactions, one result of medication error, cause around 700 deaths a year in England alone. That is about two deaths every day. When you add in other deaths to which medication error is likely to have contributed, while not necessarily being the sole cause, the number goes up to 22,000 deaths every year.[8]

The research stressed that there was no evidence that medication error rates were any lower in other countries. Indeed, international research suggests that diagnostic accuracy, one of the root causes of medication error, is normally only 90%.[9] Nearly all such errors relate to doctor–patient interaction rather than tests or referrals. The US Institute of Medicine estimated in 2015 that all of us will experience diagnostic error once in our lifetime.[10] Led by Liam Donaldson and Dr Neelam Dhingra, the WHO has therefore decided to focus on medication error as one of the major themes in its current ten-year focus on patient safety, after looking at research that suggests that it may account for 50% of all preventable harm globally, particularly when it comes to prescribing and monitoring.[11] The global cost is estimated to be $42 billion annually.[12]

There are several solutions. Much research has been done into the importance of 'differential diagnoses' – the process whereby a doctor challenges a preliminary conclusion by asking in a structured way what other explanations could account for a patient's symptoms. But when it comes to errors in the administration of medicine, the first step is more straightforward: we need to look at the data and see where mistakes are occurring.

That means linking up medication administration data with hospital admission data on a national scale, so that we understand the true scale of such harm. We also need a comprehensive audit of drug-related harms – starting with gastrointestinal bleeding, a serious condition which, if not treated, can cause significant damage. Pharmaceuticals such as non-steroidal anti-inflammatory drugs (NSAIDs), cortico-steroids, selective serotonin reuptake inhibitors (SSRIs) and antiplatelet drugs are commonly linked to gastrointestinal bleeding. Arthritis patients in particular need to know how to spot the signs of such bleeding, as they are at greater risk of experiencing it at some point, according to a US study.[13] Incorrect dosage levels or continued use of these drugs despite early signs of bleeding can all cause more serious problems.

We should also speed up the introduction of electronic prescription. While moving to electronic systems will not address every mistake, they make an obvious contribution by reducing the risk of transcription errors. They can nudge clinicians to double-check their decisions through online prompts, providing they are used sparingly, as we will see in the next chapter. Currently only about half of NHS trusts have good electronic prescription and medicines administration systems in place, so we urgently need to accelerate the introduction of these systems everywhere, as overall they have been shown to reduce prescribing errors by up to 30%.[14]

Proper human factors analysis of the root causes of medication error in primary care would probably also identify another issue we identified earlier, namely the risk that some staff are just becoming too busy to do their jobs without a high risk that mistakes will be made. According to one survey, the average GP in the UK has forty-two different patient contacts a day, a pressure that has increased post-pandemic.[15] Is it any surprise if a cancer gets missed when people are working at such pace? As ever, alleviating the risk of workforce burnout will play a major part in any solution. In the next chapter we will see how technology can also play a major role.

12
Technology

Michael Milken is the epitome of a Marmite character: a disgraced junk bond dealer whose philanthropy has saved many lives. Much of that philanthropy has centred on cancer research, following his own brush with prostate cancer after leaving prison.

He was nearly seventy when I met him to hear about that research. I found myself intrigued by a life with so many dramatic twists and turns: from a Wall Street master of the universe all the way to prison – and then to a kind of redemption. So at the end of the meeting I couldn't resist asking him what advice he would give his grandchildren as they started out on their lives. He thought for a moment and then said, 'Three things: firstly, no good deed goes unpunished; secondly, there is no first-mover advantage – only arrows in your front and back when you try to change anything; and thirdly, think about how the world is going to be, not how it is.'

At the time, I was thinking about the arrows in my own back from various changes I had been trying to make in the NHS, so his advice resonated. But perhaps the most important thing he said was the third: to think about the world as it will be, not how it is. As we wrestle with the challenge of reducing so much avoidable harm in healthcare, we must harness the bigger changes happening all around. And the biggest of those is technology.

It is a cliché to say technology changes everything – but that doesn't make it any less true. Everything, from the way we shop to the way we bank, book holidays, take exercise and listen to music, is undergoing radical change. But it has taken surprisingly long for the impact to be felt in healthcare.

For sure, we are seeing the adoption of electronic health records, standard now in American hospitals and becoming that way in the rest of the world. The NHS, often ridiculed for its backward technology, is a surprising leader in one type of electronic health record, which we will look at later, but very behind in its hospital IT systems. Most of the improvements have focused on administrative efficiency rather than patient care. In a way, this mirrors the efficiency improvements we have experienced elsewhere in our daily lives, whether it's being able to buy things without leaving the house, checking in for a flight without going to the airport or finding out tomorrow's weather without waiting for the news on TV.

But even on blindingly obvious efficiency improvements, the NHS has taken its time. When I arrived, it was reputed to be the world's biggest purchaser of fax machines, although they were in surprisingly widespread use in other countries like Germany and the United States.[1] Some GP surgeries even employed people with the title of 'Chief Fax Officer' to deal with a daily avalanche of faxes from other parts of the NHS. My immediate successor Matt Hancock, a big technology enthusiast, tried to ban the use of fax machines in the NHS entirely by March 2020 – but they were still in use when he left.[2]

Improvements in administrative efficiency ultimately allow more resources to be devoted to patient care, so they matter. But what about the direct impact technology can have on patient safety and the reduction of avoidable harm and death?

Take emergency care. A decade ago almost no emergency departments had access to GPs' electronic health records. I remember in my first year taking part in a shift in the A & E at Watford General Hospital. Lying in front of me was a woman who had been rushed in from her care home after having a fall. She was in her nineties and had dementia. She couldn't speak and was barely conscious – but what was most shocking was that the doctors knew absolutely nothing about her. They didn't know how advanced her dementia was, so had to guess why she couldn't talk: was it her dementia or her fall? They didn't even know vital information such as what medication she was on or what allergies she might have.

It was a terrible moment – but a perfectly normal one for emergency care doctors and nurses. Indeed, they are trained to make a rapid assessment based on limited information in such situations in order to give a diagnosis. Such a judgement would have been much safer, made much faster and been more accurate if they had been able to access the electronic health record from her GP surgery. It made it even more frustrating that those GP records were some of the best of their kind in the world – just unavailable when they were needed the most.

Understanding just how this happened gives important clues as to how to resolve such issues.

When Tony Blair's government introduced its Connecting for Health programme with great fanfare in 2005,[3] fiercely independent doctors in general practice decided they wanted nothing to do with it. The programme was ultimately doomed, but as it was heading for the graveyard the GP community quietly got on with their own technology transformation, appointing a small group of suppliers to develop user-friendly software programmes that allowed them to transfer patient health records from brown cardboard folders onto computers.

Over a decade, without any fanfare, this work was completed. Because in the UK the main way to access NHS services is through your GP surgery – and hospitals are required to send back reports of any care they give to the same surgery – the resulting records end up being an extremely accurate lifetime account of their patients' health. Most other countries do not use GPs as gatekeepers to the system, so do not have the opportunity to build up such a detailed record. Safely out of the hands of government, our GPs did just that – but the fruit of their work remained tantalisingly out of the grasp of the rest of the NHS for many years.

In fairness, if Blair made some unfulfilled pledges about NHS technology, so too did I, including saying in 2013 that I wanted the NHS to be 'paperless' within five years.[4] Five years away was a long time, and I didn't think for a moment I would be Health Secretary for long enough to see the pledge through. But at the start of 2018, there I still was – and the NHS was far from paperless. I knew that not least from seeing the brown cardboard folders at the end of my wife's hospital bed when our third child, Ellie, was born.

But there was progress. The person in charge of technology in the NHS was a dynamic and quirky contrarian called Tim Kelsey. To tackle issues such as those in Watford, Tim made it a priority to connect health records in GP surgeries to hospitals. Some hospitals, such as Airedale Hospital in Yorkshire, were already doing this. After a lot of prodding, the number of A & E departments able to access a version of someone's GP record rose from a handful to nearly all of them. The commitment to a paperless NHS also helped change the focus of hospitals and GPs from a rigid tradition of face-to-face delivery to a more flexible approach to patient contact, including phone and video consultations, something that was turbocharged during the pandemic. The change in approach also galvanised a vibrant med tech and health tech industry in the UK.

Technology should always be a means, and not an end in itself. While changes such as those mentioned above improved care, it was also true that some of the very best care I saw, such as by the big-hearted Dr Moran, was completely technology-free. And when implemented poorly, technology can be a barrier to the improvements in safety it is supposed to be enabling.

On a visit to San Francisco, I met someone who has thought about these issues more perhaps than anyone else. Professor Bob Wachter works for the University of California, San Francisco. His hospital is the most high-tech I have ever seen. Medicines were delivered from one end of the hospital to another by Dalek-like robots who speed silently past you, summoning lifts in advance so the doors are open before they arrive. You might have expected Wachter to be an unashamed worshipper at the technology altar – but in his seminal book *The Digital Doctor*[5] he describes just how badly things can go wrong. In it, he shows a picture by a seven-year-old girl, who was asked to draw a description of her visit to the doctor. The picture is of a man in a white coat – but instead of talking to a patient he is hunched over a computer. Perhaps it takes a seven-year-old to remind us how much, for all their efficiency, computers can be a barrier between doctor and patient.

Many doctors in the US complain that the amount of data they are required to enter into electronic health records means they barely have time to spend with patients. Wachter describes an advertisement for an emergency care doctor for a hospital in Arizona, which had 'No EHRs' (electronic health records) written at the bottom. A hospital believed it would *attract* doctors to work there, if they told them they did not keep electronic records.

Even the most obvious safety improvements made possible by technology have pitfalls. A good example is the way an electronic health record can flag potential allergies or dangerous drug reactions that a busy doctor might miss. Sodium valproate, for example, is highly effective at controlling seizures for those with epilepsy, but can do permanent damage to an unborn baby if taken while pregnant. In theory, an electronic prescribing system could flag a warning if such a drug was about to be issued to someone who was pregnant. In practice, such warnings can occasionally get lost as doctors report some systems sending them no fewer than three hundred alerts during a single working day. Not only is a vital alert missed, but the doctor's productivity is dragged right down. Some react by just switching off the alerts altogether – completely defeating the point.

Wachter did a lot of work to help NHS hospitals modernise their systems in a way that avoided such traps. His key insight was that for the benefits of new technology to translate properly into patient safety, you need systems that enhance rather than reduce the productivity of clinicians. A system designed by managers may succeed in giving them the best management information in the world – but if it means doctors spend less time with their patients, the resulting healthcare will be less safe.

None of these pitfalls, of course, should blind us to the potential of technology – or stop us trying. But to understand that potential, you must look beyond the administrative efficiencies or even things like basic safety alerts that electronic health records make possible. They are just the tip of the iceberg, because once health information becomes digitised, it becomes the building block for machine learning and genomics, both of which make many extraordinary new discoveries possible.

One of those is the ability to identify a disease before a patient shows any symptoms.

I learned about how that works from someone who isn't a doctor or a scientist, but an entrepreneur: Vinod Khosla, the billionaire co-founder of Sun Microsystems. He has shifted nearly all his investments into health innovation, as he is convinced that this is where the most dramatic changes are about to occur. He explained to me that one drop of blood has 300 biomarkers. Within a decade, he expects all of us to be sending in blood samples every few months to identify variations that could signal the start of a disease, before any external symptoms are visible.

That will allow many diseases to be diagnosed while they are still asymptomatic. We may even get to the stage when the appearance of any symptoms at all is seen as a sign of failure, because we have such high confidence in our ability to pick up cell mutations early. Khosla goes further, suggesting doctors will be cut out of diagnosis altogether: why ask a human brain to crunch the data from 300 biomarkers when a computer can do it so much more quickly?

Such changes will be extraordinary, and unlike Khosla I do not believe doctors will be written out of the process of diagnosis. But the safest way to tackle any disease will always be to destroy it before a patient shows any symptoms, and such changes are closer than many think: the NHS-Galleri cancer trial being run by King's College London and Cancer Research UK, for example, hopes to detect fifty cancers through a single blood test. A precursor to such tests is even available today: a company called Thriva receives monthly blood samples from its customers which are then analysed for things like cholesterol in a laboratory in Gloucester, with an email response sent back by a doctor within twenty-four hours.[6]

Yet the biggest way in which technology will improve the safety and quality of care is not practical but cultural. No one has thought more about this than Eric Topol, founder of the Scripps Research Translational Institute in San Diego. Topol became famous for conducting a legal battle with the American Medical Association (AMA) in 2012, to allow patients to have full access to their own medical records. The AMA argued doctors would be inhibited in what they wrote if patients could see their notes – but Topol counter-argued that it was a basic human right for patients to be able to read everything written about them. He won.

The impact of allowing patients to see their medical notes turned out to be much more radical than even he anticipated. Even though such records are barely decipherable to non-doctors when undigitised, seeing them gives patients the chance to research the medication they have been prescribed, understand potential side effects, and appreciate the importance of adherence to medicine regimes. This transfer of knowledge from doctor to patient is also a transfer of power. Responsibility for a treatment plan is then shared – as it should be – between doctor and patient rather than being solely the responsibility of a doctor. Most doctors welcome this change, quite happy to swap a pedestal for more collaborative decision-making. They know it gets results.

In his book *The Patient Will See You Now*,[7] Topol goes further: he talks about technology causing the 'democratisation of healthcare' – destroying the paternalistic, almost master–servant relationship between doctors and patients that has existed since the time of Hippocrates. Instead, the new boss is the patient. For the first time we become masters of our own healthcare destiny, seeking advice and expertise from doctors when needed, but ultimately taking our own decisions and accepting the responsibility that comes with them.

Following Topol's victory, surprising evidence emerged about immediate improvements to the safety of care. When patients in

America were given access to their medical records, they started spotting mistakes. The infallibility of doctors clearly does not extend to record-keeping. But on top of more accurate record-keeping, improved access to knowledge soon leads to improved responses to treatment from more knowledgeable patients. As Emma Hill says in an article published in the *Lancet*, 'Every patient is an expert in their own chosen field, namely themselves and their own life.'[8]

That change will be accelerated by another technological leap that is slowly becoming central to medicine: the sequencing of genomes. The first human genome was sequenced in 2003 after nearly twelve years of work and well over a billion dollars of investment. Now it is possible to sequence anyone's genome for less than $1,000 – with the cost soon likely to fall to just a few hundred dollars. Being able to understand our genetic map – and those of people in our families who have a similar genetic make-up – brings with it the possibility of everyone being able to predict the likelihood of certain diseases. A famous early example of this came when Angelina Jolie chose to have a double mastectomy after genetic profiling showed she had an 87% chance of developing breast cancer.[9]

What if you combined those two big changes?

That would mean your complete sequenced genome would sit right alongside your illness and treatment details on a digitised and comprehensive medical record. A doctor would be able to advise you prospectively, based on your genetic profile, as well as retrospectively, based on your medical history. The interaction between predictive and historic data in our individual medical records would yield extraordinary insights – both for ourselves and for everyone else, once the data is aggregated and compared. Such a change would prove to be a revolution for humanity every bit as transformative as the internet has been.

Led by people like Tim Kelsey and Noel Gordon, who ran NHS Digital for many years, the NHS has taken important steps towards this brave new world, including embracing artificial intelligence and machine learning. But it is still evolutionary rather than revolutionary change. And we have still not addressed some of the challenging ethical issues that such a revolution will force to the surface. How, for example, will we ensure that such advances are made available to everyone and not just to a wealthy few? How will we protect electronic health records from hackers?

To be true to its mission, the NHS needs to find a way of unlocking such benefits for every single citizen. It should start by declaring that, within a decade, it will decode the genome of every baby at birth. That data should then be added to a child's electronic health record in a format that allows it to be analysed and updated as we develop a better understanding of which genetic patterns lead to particular diseases. As the price of the technology falls, we should aim to roll the process out to all citizens.

Long before then, the NHS should also make it possible for all of us to access our entire medical records on an app on our phones, subject to the same kind of security we need to access bank accounts. By doing both these things, we will combine the best NHS traditions of technological innovation with equitable access – and encourage everyone to take more responsibility for their own healthcare.

But however successful such apps are, we will never see doctors replaced by computers. Writers like Yuval Noah Harari are right to predict that we will see more acceptance of the fact that the processing of large amounts of information is done more efficiently by a machine – and that algorithms can be more reliable predictors of health risks than human beings. But we will always need doctors to interpret that data, and guide their patients towards the appropriate action.

The biggest benefit for both doctors and patients should be time: more time to give and receive care and more time to develop the life-long relationships that always used to be the essence of the profession. But for patients the benefits will extend beyond more time with their doctor, beyond even extraordinary new discoveries. It will be a new sense of control: being in charge of your own health destiny in a way that has never before been possible.

PART FOUR

Making It Happen

13

Communication

Opposite me sat my biggest critic.

The meeting was somewhat easier than it might have been, because I was no longer a Cabinet minister. But if I wanted to write a book about learning from mistakes in healthcare, then I had to practise what I preached and – deep breath – listen to my own critics. I also wanted to understand how you make things happen in the NHS – and why my own efforts to do so had not always been successful. One of the most important ways you change things is by communicating effectively what you are trying to achieve. I wanted to understand how well I had done that, particularly during the bitter and damaging junior doctors' strike that lasted nearly a year.

Dr Rachel Clarke is a palliative care doctor at a hospice in Oxford. She is a former journalist and talented author. She is also a prolific tweeter – and her tweets were so hostile to me that I ended up 'unfollowing' her, for the sake of my own morale if nothing else. Her journalistic background gives her an ability to use facts and figures to deadly effect – and for many years I was the target. She agreed to meet me because, to her credit, she recognised that, whatever our differences, we had a shared commitment to patient safety. And so began a series of difficult discussions. I knew Rachel would speak her mind, and was both curious and apprehensive about what she would say.

The anger and bitterness of the strike began with a very pleasant summer, at least for me personally. David Cameron had just won an unexpected victory, and I was happy to be back at the Department of Health to pursue my passion for patient safety. We had a wonderful family holiday, with our one-year-old daughter taking her first, halting steps on a San Diego beach.

But trouble was brewing. In July, I had announced changes to doctors' contracts to improve the consistency of care at weekends.[1] I had seen data that showed a 15% increase in mortality rates for patients admitted at weekends and wanted to make changes to improve the availability of doctors. My main objective was to increase the number of consultants operating over seven days, as the evidence suggested that one of the most important things for a patient was to be reviewed early by an experienced doctor.

But I also agreed with a recommendation to change the contract for junior doctors at the same time. Ironically, given the storm these proposals would unleash, only some of the changes to that contract were about improving seven-day care. Most were long overdue productivity changes such as replacing automatic annual pay rises with merit-based awards. But such details got lost in the subsequent fog of battle.

Like me, Cameron had concerns about the consistency of seven-day care offered by the NHS, enough in fact to include it as a key pledge in our 2015 election manifesto.[2] His particular issue was not being able to get a GP appointment in the evenings or at weekends, something that was very frustrating for people who work normal office hours. I agreed with this, but was more concerned about the safety of weekend care in hospitals than the issue of convenience.

As a result, we were both up for a battle when it came to reforming contracts. Neither of us had any idea quite how big and bitter that battle would become.

The concerns I had about weekend care crystallised during a meeting I had with Frank and Janet Robinson, a couple who lost their son John partly thanks to clinical errors made on a Saturday. Because John was yet another Mid Staffs tragedy, I did not initially register the extent to which his care was impacted by a 'weekend effect'.

John was a fitness fanatic. He was six foot five, loved sport and even had his own gym at home. He had recently moved out of the family home, buying a house with his brother Clarke so he could be nearer his work as a telecommunications engineer.

One Saturday in April, John met up with a group of friends to go mountain biking in Cannock Chase. During the ride, John fell off his bike. The handlebars hit him hard in the chest and he felt excruciating pain. His friends dialled 999.

While in the ambulance, a paramedic noted down that he thought John had internal bleeding and life-threatening injuries. At the hospital he was handed over to a triage nurse. But the nurse, either not reading or ignoring the paramedic's diagnosis, parked him in a waiting room. It was the wrong call.

John lay on his own for an hour and ten minutes. He had one brief examination by a newly qualified doctor who sent him for an X-ray. No one else was consulted and it was decided John could go home with a few painkillers for some bruised ribs.

When the nurse came to tell him, John was semi-conscious and vomiting. His friends pointed this out, but the nurse said that John just needed a few more minutes. She came back with a wheelchair and a container in case John vomited again. Unable to walk, John was wheeled out to be driven home.

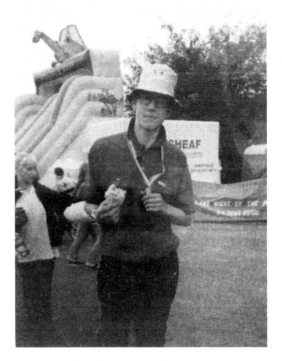

John Moore-Robinson

Sitting in my office, Frank and Janet were quite clear about why he was hurried out of the hospital: doing so meant they would hit the four-hour A & E target. Staff had been told they would face disciplinary action if they missed it, which put them under enormous pressure to discharge emergency patients quickly. But it soon became clear there was another issue in their story – the lack of a senior doctor to assess John at the weekend.

John was driven home, believing that all he needed was a good night's rest. Later that evening, the pain became so severe that he again called 999. The paramedics came round – but when he stood up to answer the door, he had lost so much blood that he had a seizure. At 1.30 a.m., John went into cardiac arrest and was transferred to the

Leicester Royal Infirmary. Resuscitation was attempted, but it was too late, because when he had fallen from his bike he had ruptured his spleen. He died shortly afterwards.

His parents knew nothing of what had happened until they got a knock on the door from two policemen. They were told that John had been rushed to the Leicester Royal, but when they arrived there they found their second son, Clarke, in a room with his fiancée Ruth, tears streaking his face. All he could say was: 'John's gone, Mum... John's gone.'

As they came to terms with the shock, Frank and Janet began to realise that something had gone badly wrong with John's care.

They found out that lots of doctors at Mid Staffs A & E were routinely taken out of 'majors' – the more serious cases – and put into 'minors', to make sure the four-hour target wasn't missed. That meant seriously ill patients were ignored. Janet says that 'following the second inquest [...] eight years after his death, we referred the triage nurse to the NMC', who informed them that the nurse 'had already been struck off the nursing register for other offences, one of which was falsifying patient discharge times from A & E and for bullying colleagues to do likewise', which she thinks is 'very telling'.

Scans, unavailable at weekends, would have shown that John had a ruptured spleen. Because it was a Saturday there was no consultant to see John, putting a huge responsibility on the shoulders of the duty junior doctor. Colliding with the handlebars of a bike is a classic cause of a ruptured spleen, which a more experienced doctor might have known but a trainee might not.

Stories such as this convinced me that things needed to change. But what did the academic evidence on the topic actually say?

A large study into the 'weekend effect', known as the Fremantle Study, concluded that the 'cohort admitted at weekend included a greater prevalence of patients with higher predicted mortality risk than those admitted during the week' and that thirty-day mortality across all admissions increases by 10% on a Saturday and 15% on a Sunday. It also said it was not possible to ascertain the extent to which these 'excess' deaths may be preventable.[3]

Other research conducted before that had said similar things. A literature review conducted by the Academy of Medical Sciences in December 2012 stated that 'there is a growing body of evidence that case mix-adjusted mortality rates are higher for patients admitted electively or as emergencies to hospital "out-of-hours", with most research focusing on weekends'.[4] Earlier, a 2010 study on weekend mortality rates by Professor Paul Aylin of Imperial College found that the 'overall adjusted odds of death for all emergency admissions was 10% higher [...] in those patients admitted at the weekend compared with patients admitted during a weekday'.[5]

In short, lots of studies had looked at this issue in the UK and around the world. Unprompted by me, the NHS had also set up its own 'Seven Days a Week Forum' to develop clinical standards to address these issues. Those standards said that patients should always be reviewed by a consultant within fourteen hours of admission to hospital – whichever day of the week they were admitted. They also said there should be seven-day access to diagnostics and certain key interventions that needed to be done by consultants.

The research seemed clear, and many senior doctors and Royal Colleges, led by NHS England medical director Bruce Keogh, had long been troubled by the issue. But how do you communicate the need for change? Predictably for a politician, I did it through a speech. I wanted to convey my determination to make changes for the benefit of patients, so the tone of the speech at the King's Fund in July 2016 was robust, perhaps over-robust.[6] The headlines reflected that, with one saying: 'Hunt goes to war with doctors'.[7]

The skirmishes started harmlessly enough, with Twitter photos posted by numerous doctors over the following weekends. They gently – and often humorously – pointed out the work that doctors already did at weekends, and all had the hashtag #ImInWorkJeremy. The humour did not last. As Rachel Clarke pointed out to me, the reason the battle was so bitter was not really the issue of weekend care itself but the context in which my request came. Concerns about staffing shortfalls were widespread. Increasing weekend cover felt to many like spreading the jam even more thinly during the week.

The result was a strike ballot, in which 98% voted in favour of strike action.[8]

But if the junior doctors were in no mood to compromise, nor was I.

It was not just the principle of weekend care that mattered to me, but also a feeling that I should not give in to some underhand tactics that had contributed to the huge majority that voted for a strike. The BMA put a 'pay calculator' on their website suggesting that the new contracts would mean pay cuts of up to 50%. When it was exposed as fiction, the calculator was quietly removed – but without any attempt to set the record straight. As Health Secretary, I had to negotiate with more trade unions than any other Cabinet minister, and felt that capitulating in the face of such tactics would send a disastrous signal.

Tactics aside, the main reason for the impasse was probably a straightforward misunderstanding about my plans – there was a serious failure in communication. Most junior doctors already worked weekends (like the junior doctor who saw John Moore-Robinson). They assumed the reason I wanted to change their contracts was to take away the few weekends they had left and pay them less for the privilege. As the people who probably work the hardest on the front line – particularly in emergency care – that made them understandably angry.

Once such misunderstandings became entrenched, they became impossible to reverse. Support for the strike grew with a series of marches and demonstrations. On one occasion, I was cycling down Whitehall after a drink with Boris Johnson. He was trying to court me for his leadership bid, which was somewhat ironic considering what was to happen four years later. Suddenly I saw a large group of demonstrators blocking the road outside the Department of Health. As I got closer, I saw their 'Save the NHS' banners and realised that they were protesting against… me. No one recognised me in my cycle helmet, and I was able to execute a lucky U-turn.

By the time the strikes actually started, positions had hardened to the extent that, while lip service was paid to a willingness to talk, no talks actually happened. Indeed, leaked WhatsApp messages revealed

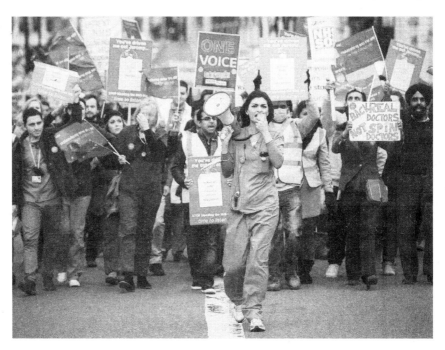

The junior doctors' strike

that the BMA had a strategy to 'draw the dispute right out' while at the same time playing a 'political game of always looking reasonable'.[9] So, with a heavy heart, I took the decision to proceed with the new contract in the hope that a demonstration of resolve would draw the matter to a close.

It did not. Reaction met counter-reaction and we ended up with more strikes, with turnout remaining high each time. I rapidly became a hate figure and I lost count of the number of times TV and radio presenters 'mistakenly' started my last name with a C rather than an H. I was also astonished by the number of Conservative Party donors who advocated taking a tough line with trade unions but wanted me to cave in, usually because they had a junior doctor son or daughter.

As the dispute ground on, I began to ask myself if I had missed something.

Were there other, genuine concerns apart from the contract that needed addressing? I asked my officials at the Department of Health to find as many areas as possible where we could address legitimate grievances. We found a number, including the inflexibility of the training process, which could wreak havoc with family life when two partners were posted in different cities.

Where we could solve a problem, we did. But there was one constant complaint that was harder to solve, namely the problem of 'rota gaps', unfilled positions on rotas because of doctor shortages. 'You claim to care about patient safety,' junior doctors seemed to be saying to me, 'so why are there all these gaps where we can't get the doctors we need to look after patients?' I had been set on getting more consultants on duty at weekends. They wanted more doctors full stop – and they had a point.

The strikes finally ended in May, after both sides were effectively bounced into talks by the Medical Royal Colleges. Somewhat to my surprise, we negotiated an agreement with the BMA leadership which had all the changes I wanted, perhaps because they were as exhausted as I was. But the mood was sufficiently sour that when the deal was put to BMA members in a ballot it was once again rejected. This time the union leadership threatened to withdraw emergency care for a full five days, which would almost certainly have led to patient deaths. I didn't believe they would follow through with it – and thankfully was proved right. The strike collapsed.

But the bitterness remained. On one level, it was the inevitable consequence of a Secretary of State refusing to compromise in tough negotiations with a union – in a dispute that became highly politicised. But given that most doctors understand there is a serious issue around seven-day care, why did it prove so difficult to communicate it?

It is partly the sheer size of the NHS. As the largest employer in Europe, it is very difficult to get messages – sometimes complex ones – across to a large, busy workforce spread throughout the country, without using the national media, which often has its own agenda. In this chapter, I want to look at the challenge of communication in more detail – because you cannot reduce avoidable harm and death without persuading other people to support you. To understand how, I consider the way communication happens in politically charged conflicts like the junior doctors' strike, but also in more everyday situations.

First, the strike. When I asked Rachel how she first heard the news about my desire to improve seven-day care, she explained that it was from a newspaper headline on her iPhone. It happened to be just before she went to bed, and reading it turned out to be a big mistake, because she then didn't sleep a wink. She interpreted the headline as a full-frontal attack on the professionalism of doctors. She found her fellow doctors equally shocked when she arrived at work the next day.

No one, of course, had read the speech, which would have given important context to the argument I was making, but as a politician you know that rarely happens. The headlines suggested that the Health Secretary thought medicine was a five-days-a-week profession. Who, doctors wondered, did I imagine delivered babies at 2 a.m.? Who did I think pieced together the broken bones of someone in a car accident at 4 a.m. on a Sunday morning? To junior doctors, some of whom had already come close to quitting because of long hours, it felt deeply insulting to be presented as money-grubbers standing in the way of better care for patients. That, of course, was the last thing I had intended, but in politics communication is everything, so you have to take responsibility for how your words are interpreted.

Rachel explained to me that junior doctors felt I was telling the public that the reason for the 'weekend effect' on mortality rates was that they were refusing to work on Saturdays and Sundays, and that I could solve this simply by changing their contract. But in reality that would not happen, because the problem was caused by a shortage of doctors – mid-week as well as at weekends. My argument was 'simply moronic' – she didn't mince her words – because it was no solution to improve services at weekends by worsening them in the week.

The result was a very heated conflict, where battle lines were drawn quickly. I am the last person who would walk across the street to pick a fight, but I found myself in the eye of a highly personal storm. For Rachel, the reason for this was straightforward: politicians who justify their actions using a mantle of principle are even more detestable than those who are 'honest' about their self-interested motives.

I don't agree with that characterisation of politicians, and my desire to improve weekend care was a sincerely held conviction. But even if many people understood that, doctors on the front line did not. To them it felt like I was trying to mask the effects of 'Tory austerity' by blaming doctors for not being prepared to work harder. I was making it an issue of contracts (their fault) instead of austerity (my fault). So

I asked Rachel how she thought I could have communicated things differently.

She said few doctors would deny that pressures and risks to care were greater at weekends, but thought I should have started by talking to people on the front line about the issue to try to win them over. Then I should have produced a financial package that increased the size of the doctor workforce. That way, as she saw it, the impetus for change would have been shared by politicians and doctors. Indeed, she thought it would have met an eager and willing response from young doctors enthusiastic to do the right thing for patients. She described junior doctors as 'the most committed workforce any CEO could hope for'.

I am not sure it would have been quite so easy. In smaller organisations, face-to-face communication builds trust, allows for nuance and means misunderstandings can be quickly sorted out. But such personal interaction is not possible with 55,000 junior doctors in 250 hospital trusts. A lot of my communication with junior doctors ended up being conducted through the national media, with its particular lens, or Facebook pages, where algorithms boosted the most inflammatory interpretations. Additionally, because there were no private talks, positions on different aspects of the dispute were taken in public, which made compromise next to impossible. The result was a dispute that lasted nearly as long as the miners' strike of 1984–85.

In politics, fights are sometimes necessary – and weekend care has improved in the NHS. We are one of the few healthcare systems to have seven-day standards and the changes I wanted to make to junior doctors' contracts were made and have been accepted. But even now many hospitals still do not meet the seven-day standards, and important changes to the contracts of more senior doctors have yet to be negotiated. But because of the miscommunication – on all sides – I paid a heavy price for winning that battle. I lost the ability to engage constructively with a key group of people on the very patient safety issues I cared about the most.

As a result, I had to spend a long time building bridges with the medical profession. It felt impossible to do that through social media, so I reverted to more traditional face-to-face visits, organising a programme of open seminars on patient safety at every NHS hospital. On one visit protesters climbed onto my car and covered it in flour; on another someone in the back row quietly unfurled a poster saying 'Your policies kill people'. But those were the exceptions, and after a year of doing such presentations the warmth of the reception increased, as did the numbers attending, often stretching to several hundred. Sadly, I was moved to the Foreign Office before I was able to get round all NHS hospitals, but I look back on that programme of visits as one of the most important things I did as Health Secretary.

The junior doctors' strike encapsulates the challenges and pitfalls of communication when it comes to a controversial issue like changing contracts. But what about when you're trying to change something everyone agrees with in the first place? That, too, can be surprisingly challenging.

One example was attempts made to address the high frequency of what surgeons call 'Never Events'. These are occurrences that the NHS classifies as wholly preventable.[10] This is because guidance is available which, if followed, should not just reduce but *eliminate* the possibility of their happening. They include such blindingly obvious mistakes as operating on the wrong part of someone's body – say, amputating the wrong foot; leaving an implement like a pair of forceps or a surgical swab inside someone after an operation; or attaching the wrong prosthetic limb to a patient.

There are around five hundred Never Events every year in the NHS.[11] About once a fortnight, tubes are incorrectly inserted through the nose or mouth when someone can't eat – potentially fatal if, for example, food ends up drip-fed into someone's lungs. Nearly once a week, someone has the wrong implant or prosthesis attached to them. And no less than twice a week do we operate on the wrong part of someone's body. While I was Health Secretary, I heard about one patient who had the wrong toe amputated, and another whose ovary was removed instead of her appendix.

I was so concerned about the issue that I put up a whiteboard on the wall in my office listing the number of Never Events by hospital for the previous week. It became the most famous whiteboard in the NHS, seen by the many doctors and managers who came to meetings with me. It was also criticised by journalists, who accused me of being more interested in NHS failures than successes. But, agree or disagree with the method, no doctor could have doubted my concern over the issue.

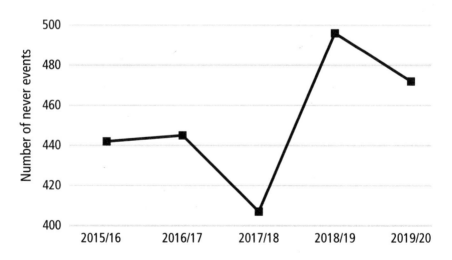

Fig. 7: Number of Never Events, 2015/16 to 2019/20 (Source: NHS England[12])

The trouble was that it was impossible to stop them. In fact, despite a big focus on surgery safety over many years, the number of Never Events may even be going up. How can that be?

Some argue the reason for the increase might be better reporting, as awareness of patient safety issues has risen. But the definition of a Never Event is pretty unambiguous compared to other types of patient harm, so while there may be some variation between reporting in different hospitals it is unlikely to be a major factor. I therefore decided to get to the bottom of the issue by commissioning an independent study from the CQC.[13] Detailed interviews were done with clinicians at eighteen trusts. The report, published after I had moved on, painted a picture that helped to explain why even blindingly obvious changes are hard to implement.

Hospitals did indeed get regular advice on how to reduce Never Events. The trouble was that this was not the only advice they were receiving. In fact, they received directions, instructions, guidance and advice from a bewilderingly large number of national organisations every week. These include messages about safety procedures from a central alert system; separate additional guidance from NHS bodies such as NHS England, NHS Improvement and the CQC; regular further guidance from professional regulators such as the GMC or the NMC; and advice from multiple professional bodies including the Royal Colleges. I asked one hospital to estimate how often they received safety-related instructions, and they totted up the number as 108 times a year.

Before you add to such instructions, it is therefore essential to put yourself in the shoes of the person receiving them – and make sure the asks are reasonable, given their other responsibilities. That means clarity about priorities and who has responsibility for implementing them. It also means, as we saw from the issue of weekend care, winning hearts and minds – because in the end, lasting change can only come from inside. The most effective communication, therefore, is not one that simply sends top-down instructions with respect to one particular issue, but one that changes the way people think. Communication should aim to change culture as much as change practice.

The CQC highlighted a good example of this in their report into Never Events. In one hospital, a nurse suspected forceps had been left inside a patient after an operation. When she told the surgeon, her concerns were dismissed out of hand. It was only after persistent nagging that they reluctantly agreed to X-ray the patient, which showed that the forceps were indeed inside the patient. They were then removed with a second operation – but the surgeon's judgement was never looked at, nor did the nurse receive any kind of apology. The culture of humility championed by brilliant thinkers like Atul Gawande was trumped by a culture of infallibility. Admitting a mistake was admitting to not being a good doctor, so better not to do it.

One of the greatest experts in getting communication right in large organisations is Professor Don Berwick, founder of the Institute for Healthcare Improvement in Boston, Massachusetts. I first met Don when he was recommended to me as someone who could write an independent report on what changes the NHS should make after Mid Staffs. His report foreshadowed many of the themes in this book. At a time when I was only really focused on the importance of transparency, Don pointed out many things I have touched on in earlier chapters, including the importance of abandoning blame as a tool for improvement, the risks of inadequate staffing and the dangers of quantitative targets. He agreed with the need for transparency – but believed that unless such transparency was communicated in a supportive context, it could fuel a destructive blame culture. It therefore needed to be conveyed as part of a bigger solution, one that placed learning and improvement at the centre of everything a healthcare organisation does. In his words, 'The NHS should continually and forever reduce patient harm by embracing wholeheartedly an ethic of learning.'[14]

Such an approach has also had many champions inside the NHS. One is Mike Durkin, who has given me much excellent advice. Another is Liam Donaldson, who has continued to advocate on patient safety issues inside the WHO after stepping down as Chief Medical Officer. One of his successors, Sally Davies, has led a global campaign on the risks of anti-microbial resistance, which is making a generation of antibiotics ineffective, a massive risk to the safety of surgery. But perhaps the most influential voice on the importance of quality and safety has been Lord Ara Darzi, who wrote a seminal report on the importance of high-quality care when he was a health minister in a previous Labour government.[15] Ara is an eminent former surgeon who had a brief stint on the political front line. When I got to know him subsequently, I came to have a deep respect for his heartfelt commitment to maintaining the highest standards of care.

More instructive, however, are local champions who have shown in their own organisations how it is possible to communicate safety improvements in a way that changes not just practice but culture as well. We have heard about Marianne Griffiths at Western Sussex, Clare Panniker at Basildon and Gary Kaplan at Virginia Mason. But the chief executive who first helped me understand this was Sir David Dalton, who at the time was chief executive at Salford Royal NHS Foundation Trust. Like the others, David is surprisingly modest and softly spoken. But his quiet style of leadership was one of the most effective I ever saw.

Back in 2007 – precisely when the events at Mid Staffs were unfolding – David travelled to Boston to attend a seminar on patient safety.

He felt somewhat inadequate, because he realised he knew so little about it despite running a large hospital. So on his return he asked his team how much patient harm there actually was at Salford Royal.

The answer came back: they did not know. No one had ever asked before. So he asked them to analyse the harms they knew about – such as pressure ulcers, infections and falls. They knew their hospital mortality rate was about the national average, but concluded that on top of this there were around 850 instances of avoidable harm every month in the hospital.

Ignoring the pressure from the system to focus on national targets, he and his team put together the first quality improvement programme in the NHS with a specific focus on reducing harm and saving lives. His objective was to save 1,000 lives in three years – or as he put it to staff, the equivalent of eight double-decker loads of bus passengers.[16]

Rather than taking the command-and-control approach that was fashionable at the time, he encouraged staff to come up with their own ideas. Those ideas were rigorously tested – and were implemented across the whole hospital only if they had a measurable effect. He didn't even make the decisions about which improvements to roll out himself, but left that decision to a representative cross-section of staff who were organised into a 'learning collaborative'. As he says, power is not a zero-sum game: 'The more you give away the more you get back.' He backed up this new engagement by spending – with his executive team – at least half a day a month working alongside staff on the front line.

But it wasn't just staff he wanted to listen to – it was patients too.

David describes how a young man died in his hospital after not responding to treatment. It turned out the man's mother had warned clinical staff he was deteriorating, but had not been listened to. So the hospital set up a family helpline, which to this day allows families instant access to a senior nurse in another part of the hospital if they think their concerns are not being addressed.

Behind these changes, he also championed a much more scientific use of data. Most hospital board papers provide aggregated performance data – but David realised those numbers concealed large variations in performance between different units and wards. So he made sure the data revealed not just the hospital average but data for each ward and department. By focusing relentlessly on variation he was able to establish where best practice was happening – and where improvements needed to be made.

Safer care saves money. So David decided to do something else. He invested the hospital's financial surplus into staff training on quality improvement. He also improved morale by replacing the majority of his clinical directors – high-ego consultants of the traditional kind – with a younger generation of doctors, picked not for the length of their experience but for their skill as team players.

The result was dramatic changes – not just to the safety of patient care, but to the culture of the organisation. Salford Royal received the top rating for quality from the CQC for four consecutive years and became the first acute trust in the country to get the coveted 'outstanding' rating.[17] It reduced C. diff infections by 95% and eliminated MRSA. It completely stopped patients acquiring the worst types of pressure ulcers, and screens every patient for sepsis when they arrive at A & E. Its mortality rates are among the lowest in the country.

David then took over the running of some neighbouring hospitals that were in difficulty. One of them, Oldham Hospital, was closely involved in the response to the Manchester Arena terror attack. I went to thank staff there for their help counselling bereaved families. The chief nurse, Elaine Inglesby-Burke, was another remarkable leader who exuded both compassion and authority. She explained to me the difficulty of their work – how do you counsel a family whose child's body has been blown up into a hundred pieces? After listening to them I found my eyes welling up, and soon all of us in that small room – Elaine included – were sobbing away.

Seeing the innate humility and humanity of people like David and Elaine made me ask why it is that in large and complex organisations the best leaders are often not those with the biggest presence. Such leaders have succeeded, among other reasons, because they are more likely to assemble strong leadership teams around them, rather than being louder characters who tend to be surrounded by yes-men. In *Good to Great*, Jim Collins calls this 'level five leadership' – the ability to show a combination of both humility and fierce resolve.

And you need both qualities if you are to communicate effectively. Fierce resolve is necessary in any leader, because people need to know their boss has the strength of character to overcome the many obstacles they face. But humility matters because unless they feel listened to people will just take orders rather than thinking for themselves. Organisations that reduce avoidable harm and death nurture constant curiosity in their teams about whether there is a safer or better way – and give them the autonomy to try out new approaches. Only when you communicate as much by listening as by talking can you harness the inner genius of everyone in an organisation.

The NHS has a budget bigger than the GDP of most countries in the world – indeed, if it were a country in its own right it would be the 33rd largest, ahead of Hungary, Morocco and Sri Lanka.[18] Is it just too big to run? Or at least too big to communicate complex but important messages effectively? Probably yes, at least if you adopt a command-and-control approach to getting messages across. But if you understand that the best communication seeks to empower rather than direct, anything is possible.

14

Zero

Joe Rafferty is the quietest and most reflective NHS chief executive I have ever met. He speaks in a soft Irish voice. A former doctor, he has spent most of his life in NHS management. He now runs Mersey Care NHS Foundation Trust, with responsibility for mental health provision across most of Merseyside, including the city of Liverpool.

After he became chief executive in 2012, one of Joe's hospital units had two suicides in just six months. They investigated what had happened and put in place additional safety measures. Then the unthinkable occurred – a third suicide. Joe and his team were shocked to the core. Coming on the heels of the previous tragedies, they asked themselves if they really were learning when things went wrong. Did they have a culture of prevention or reaction?

Joe had previously met a charismatic city leader from Detroit called Ed Coffey, someone I have also met. Coffey is famous for pioneering a controversial 'zero suicide' strategy in the city, which had cut suicides dramatically. He also pioneered the term 'perfect depression care' to capture the psychological as well as physical needs that affect many people with long-term physical conditions such as diabetes or a heart condition. Joe asked himself whether this kind of holistic care, including the bold ambition of 'zero suicide', was something an NHS mental health service could aim for.

Some of his staff were suspicious: was it another target to beat them up with when they failed? Joe was clear from the outset that any strategy should not be a target but a means to encourage staff to be ambitious.

Any mental health organisation knows you can reduce suicide with practical measures, so that's where Joe and his team started. They removed 'ligature' points – sharp corners such as hooks or window handles to which cords or bed sheets could be attached. They then arranged the wards so that nurses always had a clear line of sight to every patient. They also looked at less tangible but equally important measures, such as reducing staff turnover so that staff and patients got to know each other better.

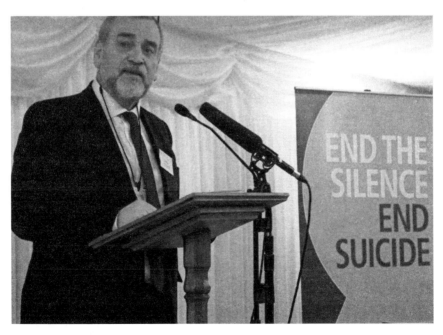

Joe Rafferty

But sometimes the best of intentions make things worse.

If your objective is zero suicides and someone tries to kill themselves with a belt, you could ban belts. You might guarantee there will not be a repeat, but as Joe says, everyone's trousers will be loose and then where is the dignity for patients? Likewise, if someone attaches a cord to the back of a bathroom door, you can remove the doors to bathrooms. Again, it guarantees no repeat – but also no privacy. If you wanted to take even more extreme measures you could eliminate suicide altogether by sedating higher-risk patients – something no one would advocate these days.

Joe realised that a compliance mentality that led to 'ticking a box' would miss the point. He needed a better way.

Working with his team, he soon realised that the most effective way to lower the risk of suicide was not just practical steps but actively working to reduce tension and conflict. That meant focusing on reducing a patient's underlying distress. The result was that they started to take a very different view of much common practice in psychiatric wards, including procedures such as holding people down by force when they were on the point of violence (known as 'restraint', which we came across in the 'homecare' chapter) or locking people up in a room on their own (known as 'seclusion'). Both practices address a short-term safety issue but can raise risk in the longer term.

One of Joe's patients was a lady who as a child had been abused by a sex ring she called the 'uncles'. She had had an abortion at the age of twelve and had tried to kill herself on multiple occasions. After she was restrained on one occasion, she asked to speak to a consultant. 'When I'm being held down, I don't see my adult hands, I see my five-year-old hands. The people pressing down on me aren't nurses, they are my abusers.' Joe realised that far from reducing tension, the act of restraint was re-traumatising her.

239

So Mersey Care set about training staff to de-escalate difficult situations without using restraint, the use of which they reduced by half over a year.[1] Another mental health trust in Gloucestershire actually eliminated the practice of seclusion altogether. They were prompted to do it because they happened to run out of space, but rather than trying to find a new room to lock people up in, they decided to train staff in de-escalation so they could end the practice completely. The benefits of such changes accrue to staff as much as patients: by reducing tension, Joe halved assaults on staff over just a year.

There are eighty inpatient suicides every year in the NHS and, inspired by Joe's story, I persuaded the NHS to adopt its own zero suicide aim for all patients admitted to mental health units.[2] It was a controversial thing to do. As with Joe's staff at Mersey Care, I came across many psychiatrists who worried I was setting an aim that was impossible to achieve. But I was given strong support and encouragement by Tim Kendall, whom we came across earlier, and together we set about trying to win the argument with the psychiatrist community. Joe went even further with Mersey Care, embracing zero suicide as an objective for *all* patients, including those living in the community. We restricted our new ambition to inpatients, because of the risk of the unintended consequence that less experienced chief executives than Joe might react by slowing down discharges into the community.

But even with patients living in their own homes, Joe showed that a zero suicide ambition was not impossible. Mersey Care realised it was particularly important for community patients to have a good crisis response, so they set up liaison psychiatry teams able to spring into action at any time of the day or night. Joe made sure the trust had properly staffed outreach teams so they could follow up patients early after they were discharged, when they observed that the risks were highest. He also worked hard with his local A & E departments to make sure they were able to offer proper care to people who arrived with a mental health crisis, particularly if they were self-harming. Finally, he reduced the time people waited for treatment after they were assessed, because research showed a heightened suicide risk in the period between assessment and first treatment.

The changes worked. There was a 90% reduction in the number of patients returning to A & E with self-harm and big improvements in the satisfaction levels of patients with depression or anxiety. Most importantly, for over three years they did not have a single suicide in the week after a patient was discharged. Mersey Care reduced its suicides by one third, double the decline nationally. Their efforts have saved sixteen lives to date.[3]

What is the secret of Mersey Care's success? Joe says it is as much about the way staff are treated as how patients are looked after. He has worked hard to replace a blame culture with the 'just culture' we looked at earlier. Most organisations try to address failures through increasing the accountability of staff for things that have gone wrong. But Joe says you need 'prospective accountability' for reducing harm in the future, as much as 'retrospective accountability' for harm that has happened. As the airline pilot Martin Bromiley would say, it is not about who is to blame but what is to blame. It is a different but equally hard-edged accountability to learn from mistakes, which involves changing not just practice but also the mindset. Insisting on WHO checklists before operations can lead to dramatic improvements – but Joe believes they will tend to plateau, unless you also change the way people think.

In this section, we will examine how to make change happen in large organisations. When it comes to preventable harm and death, is it sensible or counter-productive to 'aim for zero'? Some say there will always be a certain level of harm. Others, like Joe, ask a different question: if the number is not zero, what level of harm is acceptable?

241

Joe asked that question with respect to suicide, of which there are five to six thousand cases every year in England and Wales.[4] But exactly the same question could be applied to Never Events, medication error, failing to spot sepsis or any other type of patient harm. But to its credit, mental health care has progressed furthest in questioning whether we should ever compromise our ambitions by aiming for less than zero.

Steve Mallen was a City high-flyer who had never worked in the NHS or indeed the public sector. Around the same age as Joe, his career could not have been more different. He worked for a well-known property company and flew around the world setting up overseas offices and advising multinational corporations. Home for him was near Cambridge, where he was happily married with three lovely children. Or at least, it *was* a happy family – until his eighteen-year-old son Edward took his own life.[5]

When I met Steve, he had the weathered face of someone who has lived a thousand lives. There was none of the smooth confidence associated with jet-setting businessmen. But there was a different type of confidence: a steely belief that effective campaigning could and would prevent Edward's tragedy being repeated. And a total and utter determination to make that happen.

He told me that Edward, too, was on track to be a high-flyer. He had a place at Cambridge, where his father had been a student. His CV was impeccable: head boy at both his primary and secondary schools, a gifted classical pianist, a cricketer, good friends – and voted by his schoolmates the person most likely of all of them to become prime minister. It was, I reflected, uncannily similar to my own life at that age – a loving, middle-class family, confidence bred from success and high hopes for the future.

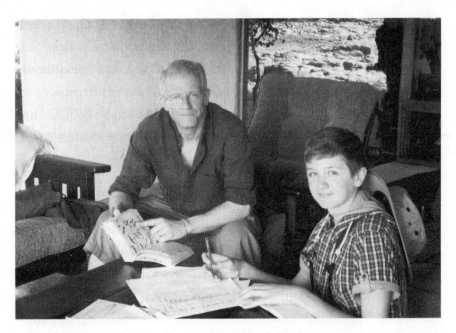

Edward on holiday with his father Steve

But then things changed. As can happen with mental illness, there was no apparent trigger. Over a period of about eight weeks, Edward was gripped by severe depression. He started to withdraw from the things he enjoyed. The piano-playing stopped. But because he had no history of mental health problems, the family were not prepared. Steve says it felt like Edward had contracted lung cancer without having smoked a single cigarette.

Edward went to see his GP, a family friend, and was referred to the local mental health service as an emergency suicide risk. Unfortunately, the nurse who assessed him was only in his second week of unsupervised work. Edward's polite and intelligent persona and seemingly safe family setting led to his case being downgraded to 'routine'. That meant he would have to wait between six and nine months for a therapy appointment.

Instead, he was given a couple of websites to look at. But his medical notes were never completed and there was no communication back to his GP. In fact, by the time he died, Edward had told five different medical professionals that he was actively thinking of taking his own life. Twice, he said he would be happy for his parents to be informed about his condition and involved in his care. But nobody told his parents a thing.

Then, on a cold, bright February afternoon, four police officers arrived at Steve's front door to tell him that Edward had killed himself just yards away from their house.

As his dad described it to me, Edward 'played' all of the music at his own funeral, as it came from remastered recordings put together by his friends. Against advice from many, at one point in the service Steve stood next to his son's coffin and made a solemn public promise to his dead son: he would investigate his untimely death and seek reforms to mental health provision so that no other family would go through the same agony.

In trying to ease Steve's pain, many suggested that Edward's death had been a terrible accident which nobody could have averted. But when he researched the subject, it became clear Edward's death could have been prevented. An independent investigation and a coroner's report later came to the same conclusion.

People like Edward die every day, Steve reminded me softly. A man takes his own life in England and Wales every two hours[6] and one third are in contact with their local mental health services. Another third have been to see their GP in the previous year.[7]

A particular focus of Steve's campaigning has been the disparity in care between mental and physical health, which Steve noticed after he was unlucky enough to be viciously assaulted in an unrelated incident. He was inundated with help – from the police, from the NHS, the criminal justice system and victim support groups. Conversely, when Edward died they received little support – just a couple of website addresses left behind by the police on a scrap of paper. Thanks to Steve's campaigning, that is starting to change.

Steve met Joe Rafferty at a conference in Belfast, and together with the senior psychiatrist Geraldine Strathdee they set up the Zero Suicide Alliance.[8] It focuses on spreading best practice and a just culture across the NHS to reduce the national suicide rate. It now has a membership base of nearly 400 organisations comprising around 250 NHS trusts, commissioners and Public Health Directorates and more than 100 private sector organisations. Every single member aims not just to reduce suicide, but to eliminate it. They have, however, recently been told their public funding will be cut, a terrible decision I hope will be reversed.

'I am simply a father honouring a promise to my beloved son,' Steve told me. How will he know if that promise has been fulfilled? 'I just need to know that if someone like Edward were to walk into a mental health facility today, the outcome would be different. We are nowhere near this, but the tide has turned.'

Prior to meeting Steve, I had met other determined patient campaigners, such as Ken Lownds, who advocated a zero harm approach. Joe, however, was the first health leader I met who was prepared to challenge the orthodoxy in medicine that some level of harm is inevitable or acceptable. In the US, I also met an inspiring and committed entrepreneur called Joe Kiani in 2018, who had founded a movement to do exactly the same, the Patient Safety Movement. Their efforts, alongside the Zero Suicide Alliance, make a refreshing contrast to my early briefings as Health Secretary, when I was told that a 10% harm rate for patients was simply the 'cost of doing business'.

In practice, of course, zero harm is unlikely to be reached. That is partly because the goalposts move with advances in technology and our understanding of medicine, making events that would previously have been considered inevitable newly 'preventable'. For that reason, 'zero harm' should always be an ambition rather than a formal target. But if we reject it as an ambition, our actions are destined to fall short of the potential for change. Hence the title *Zero* for this book. As in the apocryphal saying by Aristotle, the problem is not aiming too high and missing a goal – but aiming too low and hitting it.

Ultimately, though, aiming for zero preventable harm is more than a tactic to raise ambition – it is also a statement of values. It is saying, quite simply, that every patient in your care will be treated as well as if they were your own mother, father, son or daughter. Every single avoidable death should be treated with the seriousness with which each of us would treat a family loss. Isn't that what medicine has always stood for?

15

Patient Power

Whatever changes need to be made in modern healthcare systems to reduce avoidable harm and death, the biggest difference of all can be made not by politicians or doctors but by patients. No one has more impact on our health than we do ourselves.

That is because even if every single change I suggest in this book were implemented, things would still go wrong unless we as patients take responsibility for our side of the bargain. Sally Davies says that less than 15% of our health is accounted for by the healthcare we receive,[1] a statistic that is normally used to encourage people to lead healthier lifestyles. But personal responsibility also matters if we want to reduce the likelihood of medical error affecting our care.

Technology is making that easier. As Eric Topol has shown, access to our own medical records is changing the balance of power between patients and doctors by putting people in the driving seat when it comes to their own health. Being able to access medical records online, as I would like all NHS patients in England to be able to do, will give us all the chance to find out much more about the medicines we are taking and properly understand any diagnosis. Instead of simply following instructions, we can turn ourselves into an expert patient, an equal partner with the doctor.

Approaching treatment this way makes it far more likely to be successful, not just because patients will then understand why recommendations are being made, but because they can actively help their medical team reduce the risk of harm. That is one of the reasons why St Thomas' Hospital in London, where my mother used to be a nurse, now plays an airline-style safety video to every overnight patient at the start of their stay.

Contrary to what many expect, doctors also welcome the chance to have discussions with more knowledgeable patients. They would prefer an informed to an uninformed patient, because it increases the likelihood of success. Such patients are more likely to stick to complicated medicine regimes and more likely to make recommended lifestyle changes. Changing the balance of power between doctor and patient therefore becomes an opportunity, rather than a threat to professional status.

But this book also reveals what most health professionals – but few patients – know: there is a large and indefensible variation in the quality and safety of care between different NHS organisations. Some are truly among the best in the world, but others have a long way to go. Often, the quality and safety of that care has surprisingly little to do with how old the buildings are – outstanding care can sometimes be delivered from a portacabin a few miles away from a gleaming new PFI hospital in special measures. So as well as finding out more about your disease or condition, it is vital to learn more about the organisation delivering your care. England remains the only country in the world where detailed, independent reports are available publicly, full of objective analysis of the safety and quality of care in every hospital, and even in the departments within a hospital, one of the key reforms introduced after Mid Staffs.

	CQC rating					
Provider name	Overall	Safe	Effective	Well led	Responsive	Caring
Barts Health NHS Trust	Requires improvement	Requires improvement	Good	Good	Requires improvement	Good
Bedfordshire Hospitals NHS Foundation Trust	Good	Requires improvement	Good	Good	Outstanding	Good
Barking, Havering and Redbridge University Hospitals NHS Trust	Requires improvement	Requires improvement	Good	Good	Requires improvement	Good
Cambridge University Hospitals NHS Foundation Trust	Good	Good	Good	Good	Requires improvement	Outstanding
Bolton NHS Foundation Trust	Good	Good	Good	Outstanding	Good	Good
Chelsea and Westminster Hospital NHS Foundation Trust	Good	Good	Good	Outstanding	Good	Good

Table 5: Examples of recent trust ratings data (Source: CQC[2])

Such data should always be treated with care. Hospitals are large organisations, and there are huge variations *inside* them as well as between neighbouring hospitals. There will always be plenty of examples of outstanding care at hospitals with low ratings – as well as, sadly, poor care at hospitals with good ratings. Individual surgeon outcomes should always be adjusted for case mix, so that doctors who take on more risky cases are not penalised. But understanding the limits of such data does not make it wrong – and the more we, as patients, use it, the more doctors and hospitals will sit up and take note of what it says. Used wisely, patient power makes care safer for everyone.

Sometimes, alas, things will go wrong – even for the best-informed patients in the best-run hospital. Here there is another important lesson from the often distressing stories in this book: if you sense something is not right with the care you or a loved one is receiving, speak out. Nearly every story we have come across has a moment when a grieving relative realised they could have made a crucial intervention that might have saved the life of a loved one. Sometimes traditional British deference makes people nervous about 'causing a fuss', but as Melissa Mead says, usually a parent's instinct about a child is right – and the same is true for all loved ones. However good the care provided by frontline professionals is, they can never know a patient as well as their own families can. It isn't just doctors and nurses who need to speak out – patients and families must too.

That is even more important in the aftermath of a tragedy, however painful and difficult it might be. This book is a tribute to the many families who have done just that and campaigned publicly for change. But there are many others too, including some who may have approached me unsuccessfully during my time as Health Secretary. Ben Condon's father Allyn is one of those, and I apologise to him and anyone else who did not get the attention or response they deserved from me during my time in office. All such families have endured the most heartbreaking loss. All could have reacted in a more 'normal' way – private grieving, followed by a painful attempt to 'move on'. But in every case they chose a harder path, deciding to relive their agony over and over again in order to force change.

Surprisingly often, they succeed.

The Mid Staffs enquiry demanded by Deb Hazeldine, Julie Bailey and others led to 290 recommendations, most of which have been enacted. Without it there would have been no new independent inspection regime for NHS hospitals and surgeries.

The Kirkup Inquiry set up as a result of James Titcombe's campaigning has not had all its recommendations implemented. But it did lead to the setting up of the world's first independent investigatory body modelled on what happens after airline crashes, for which James Titcombe now works. Called the Healthcare Safety Investigations Branch, it was initially led by someone who previously ran the Air Accidents Investigation Branch (AAIB) for the airline industry.

Sara Ryan's campaigning after the death of her son Connor led to the Learning from Deaths programme, requiring all hospitals to have structured processes to examine and learn from unexpected deaths. Although that programme has now been wound up, the Department of Health claims that is because such systems are now in place. Hospitals also have a legal requirement to publish estimates of their own levels of avoidable death, something that is not happening as consistently as it should but has made a difference. It also prompted the government to implement the Medical Examiner programme, meaning that each hospital death is independently checked by a second doctor.

The American thinker Margaret Mead is thought to have said: 'Never doubt that a small group of thoughtful, committed people can change the world. Indeed, it's the only thing that ever has.' All of these families have proved her right.

It was also a privilege for me as a politician to meet such campaigners. Time and time again, I found myself marvelling at their courage, their determination and their decency. None of them ever wanted financial compensation – just to stop other families experiencing the torture they had endured. Whatever mistakes I may have made, they kept me honest – or, as Marianne Griffiths might say, gave me my 'true north'.

But the uncomfortable reality is that their job will never end. When I left the Department of Health after six years of focusing on the issue of avoidable harm and death, there were still three outstanding inquiries.

The first concerned 456 deaths at Gosport War Memorial Hospital caused by the routine over-prescription of drugs. These non-recent cases are now being investigated by the police. Families had to campaign for more than twenty years before the terrible truth emerged that the deaths of their loved ones were indeed not 'natural'. As with so many other stories in this book, many of those deaths might not have happened if the establishment had listened when junior NHS staff and relatives spoke out about their concerns, instead of treating them as troublemakers.

The Gosport Independent Panel was led by Bishop James Jones, an extraordinarily humble and compassionate man who also led the Hillsborough Independent Panel. He memorably accused the authorities of displaying the 'patronising disposition of unaccountable power'. Sadly, he went on to discover exactly the same thing at Gosport. Never have I met someone more willing to speak truth to power.

The second outstanding inquiry was being conducted by former Health Minister Julia Cumberlege, into the use of certain treatments for women – a pregnancy test now discontinued, an epilepsy drug that is highly dangerous for pregnant women to take, and the use of surgical vaginal mesh which can cause permanent and extremely painful damage. In each case, it appears that, at a very minimum, there was no mechanism for patients to express concerns about the unintended side effects of their treatments. Thanks to her report, now published, the government has agreed to establish a Patient Safety Commissioner.[3]

The third outstanding inquiry was into maternity deaths at Shrewsbury and Telford Hospital NHS Trust. I agreed to set up that inquiry after meeting Rhiannon Davies and Richard Stanton, who were devastated by the death of their daughter Kate. Led by Donna Ockenden, an experienced and tenacious NHS leader with a background in midwifery, it started by looking at twenty-three deaths. By the time her final report was published in 2022 it had increased to nearly 1,500 cases. She concluded after careful independent examination that nine mothers and over 200 babies might have survived with better care. She talked about a culture of refusing to listen to families that lasted over two decades with mothers being blamed, sometimes for their own deaths. The NHS has now agreed no mother should be put under pressure to have a 'natural birth' when a Caesarean section would be safer.[4]

There will always be tragedies in healthcare, so there will be many inquiries to come, not least the independent public inquiry the government has announced into the handling of the Covid-19 pandemic. The question is not just whether such reports gather dust, but why are they necessary in the first place? We put it on the shoulders of grieving relatives to push for change, instead of building a system hungry to make such changes automatically. If we addressed the issues around workforce shortages and workplace culture, notably replacing a blame culture with a learning culture, we could free up thousands of committed doctors and nurses to advocate and implement change without the need to put families through such torture.

The stories in this book are mainly from the UK, but campaigning to reduce avoidable harm in healthcare is now happening across the world. After I moved from the Department of Health to the Foreign Office, I couldn't shake the patient safety bug, and worked with my former health colleagues to petition the WHO to highlight its importance by having an annual patient safety day. World Patient Safety Day now happens on 17 September every year, and in 2021 was championed in eighty-nine countries, with 130 monuments illuminated in orange to mark the day.

To his credit, even when he was busy during the pandemic, WHO Director General Tedros Adhanom Ghebreyesus has shown great

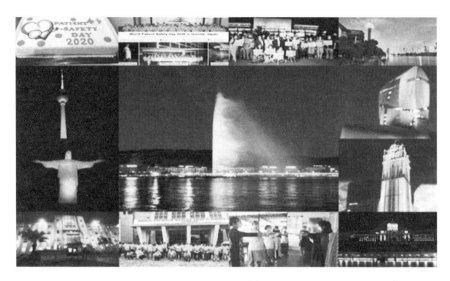

Monuments and landmarks lit in orange for World Patient Safety Day

personal commitment to patient safety. He decided that the 2020s should be a global 'decade of patient safety'.[5] With five preventable deaths every minute, he believes the time has come to address the medical error that is responsible for more deaths across the world than tuberculosis and malaria combined.[6] As a result, nearly all the stories in this book have echoed around conference rooms in the WHO headquarters in Geneva at different moments in the last few years.

So what does all this mean for the future of the NHS?

Some people have asked whether knowing in such depth what can go wrong has changed my view of it. I certainly came to understand the reality that we make mistakes – sometimes terrible ones – and tolerate a totally unacceptable level of variation in quality of care. But I also came to believe that if it wanted to be, the NHS could become the safest, highest quality healthcare system in the world. Why?

Partly because over the long period I was Health Secretary, I never once met any resistance to the idea that we should do more to reduce and eliminate avoidable deaths. On the contrary, I realised that patient harm troubled doctors, nurses, midwives and managers every bit as much as it troubled me. Indeed, the global movement to reduce harm in healthcare had much UK participation long before I became Health Secretary, including from the former health minister Lord Ara Darzi and the former Chief Medical Officer Liam Donaldson.

While we should never turn our backs on the innovation you get in some private systems, I also came to realise that, for all its bureaucracy, the NHS has some important advantages too. Whether it is improving cancer survival rates, diagnosing dementia or indeed eliminating preventable deaths, it is much easier to unite people around a simple patient-focused goal when there are no shareholders. That is one reason why I have always believed the NHS should remain a public service.

But it has practical advantages too. Uniquely among major healthcare systems, it can collect and share data easily. This makes silo-busting programmes like Tim Briggs's GIRFT much easier to deliver. Central structures can be frustrating, but they should make standardisation of practice and the elimination of variation easier than in diffuse systems – at least in theory.

The NHS can also set an example. For all its failings, it has a unique global reach and continues to exert a fascination well beyond our shores. Even though it continues to be demonised as 'socialised medicine' in some parts of the American political spectrum, many clinicians from the US look with envy at a system able to deliver high-quality care to the poorest patients without sending them an invoice. That global interest in the NHS means that if it chooses to blaze a trail on patient safety, it will save lives not just in the UK but across the world.

At the same time, we must always remain open to learning from other countries. We discussed the way Virginia Mason in Seattle has improved safety by dismantling hierarchies, but there are many other examples of good practice, including the prevention models used by Kaiser Permanente or GroupHEALTH in the US, and the surgery safety achieved by Apollo in India. We should also learn from whole systems overseas, whether from Sweden for maternity safety, South Korea for pandemic preparedness or New Zealand for no-fault compensation.

The way to make sure we embed learning from best practice either at home or abroad is to make sure our national debate, in this crucial post-pandemic period, is focused not just on money and manpower, but also on culture. Plenty of places inside the NHS show the miracles that are possible when you get the culture right, even against a backdrop of tight resources and capacity. I've written about Salford Royal, Mersey Care and Western Sussex but there are many more examples across the NHS and care system I have not had space to write about.

The noble ideas that led to the founding of the NHS are based on the idea of equality: that every citizen, rich or poor, young or old, living in a city or in the countryside, has the same value – and that as a result all should be able to access healthcare, irrespective of the size of their bank account. Now, in the wake of a horrific pandemic, we face a moment of choice: we can moderate our ambitions in the face of the many challenges ahead – or rise to the moment as our forebears did after the Second World War. I hope we choose the latter and turn this into a '1948 moment'. We have built the most accessible healthcare system in the world – let's make it the safest and highest quality as well.

Doing so will save enormous sums of money, a worthwhile objective. But the main reason is not financial. It's ethical: in rejecting outright the idea that any tragedy is 'inevitable' or the 'price of doing business' we are building a healthcare system in which every single patient matters.

If you, too, want to change the culture to tackle the scourge of avoidable harm, why not be part of the movement for change? Write to your elected representative or join a patient safety or patient rights organisation. The WHO Patients for Patient Safety network now has over 250 members spread across 52 countries and can be contacted by email at pfps@who.int.

Things are starting to move in the right direction, and you will not be alone.

POSTSCRIPT

This book has actually been seven years in the making. In July 2015, I decided to write a book telling the stories of some of the patients and families I had met as Health Secretary. As a Cabinet minister, I sought special permission from the Cabinet Office to publish a book, which was generously agreed. I started interviewing people I had met or heard about but then got caught up in a succession of 'events' – winter crises, money shortages and strikes – that meant I was not able to finish the book until after I had left the government in 2019. Almost as soon as I had completed a first draft the pandemic struck, which caused further delays. But three lockdowns also gave me a chance to think through and test the arguments I wanted to make.

As this book was going to print, Donna Ockenden's report into the most horrific maternity scandal at Shrewsbury and Telford hospital trust was published. It will, I believe, be as seminal as the Francis Inquiry into Mid Staffs. The fact that such a damning report should come out, even after so much effort in recent years on patient safety, demonstrates both how difficult it is to change culture and how important it is to keep trying.

Many people have helped me write this book in addition to the patients and families who were my original inspiration. Matthew Richardson wrote up many of the original interviews. Rafael Kochaj and Adam Smith did a huge amount of vital research and Adam is now doing a wonderful and committed job running Patient Safety Watch. My agent Jonny Geller helped me to keep faith with the project in its early, vulnerable days, while never shying away from penetrating challenge. My publisher Mark Richards filled me with enthusiasm exactly when I needed it. My editor Jack Ramm immediately understood what I was trying to do and thoughtfully helped me structure the book and arguments in a far more logical way. My copy-editor Gesche Ipsen has the kind of eagle eye for detail I can only dream of and was a huge pleasure to work with. Alex Billington did a brilliant perfectionist's job laying out the book and Elspeth McPherson was amazingly patient during my amateur reading of the audio book.

Sue Beeby, Christina Robinson, Paul Harrison and Ed Jones were the fantastic special advisers (spads) who came with me on the journey and have continued to be a source of wise (and sometimes frank) advice. Spads sometimes get a bad press, but I have never worked with a team of people smarter or more decent.

I also need to thank the two Prime Ministers who chose me to be Health Secretary. David Cameron was always passionately and personally committed to the NHS following his own family experiences. He backed me against considerable opposition in one of the three most important decisions I took on patient safety, namely to introduce a legally independent inspection regime for hospitals. Theresa May equally supported me, despite the many other pressures she was going through, on the other two big decisions: to make historic increases in the number of doctors, nurses and midwives we train and to give the NHS the biggest single budget increase in its history. I had many excellent ministers supporting me over the years too, and although I can't mention them all I must credit Philip Dunne for his calm and wise counsel and Steve Brine for his personal commitment to improving cancer treatment. Most of all I must thank my wife Lucia for tolerating with great humour both a politician husband (never much fun) and an amateur writer who locked himself away for long stretches.

All royalties from this book will go to Patient Safety Watch, a small charity I set up to fund research by Imperial College into patient safety issues. The first fruits of that work will be published shortly after this book and I am enormously grateful to Ara Darzi and his team at Imperial for making that collaboration possible.

NOTES

Introduction

1   Aneurin Bevan as quoted in BBC, *Enquiry – Portrait of a GP*, 10 February 1965, https://www.bbc.co.uk/archive/enquiry--portrait-of-a-gp/z4xf2sg

2   Jennifer Newton, 'Britons reveal the top 50 things that make them proud to be British', *Daily Mail*, 2 April 2020, https://www.dailymail.co.uk/travel/travel_news/article-8180151/Britons-reveal-50-things-make-proud-British-NHS-David-Attenborough.html; Polly Hudson and Rhian Lubin, 'Top 50 reasons we're proud to be British', *Daily Mirror*, 16 September 2016, https://www.mirror.co.uk/news/uk-news/top-50-reasons-were-proud-8853346

3   New Zealand's Social Security Act 1938 paved the way for its universal healthcare system to be put in place. The National Health Service Act 1946 came into effect in 1948 to establish our NHS.

4   According to a survey by NHS Providers, 92% of trusts have concerns about staff well-being, stress and burnout following the pandemic: 'The impact of the pandemic on the workforce', 30 June 2020, https://nhsproviders.org/recovery-position-what-next-for-the-nhs/the-impact-of-the-pandemic-on-the-workforce

5   Eric C. Schneider et al., 'Mirror, mirror 2017: international comparison reflects flaws and opportunities for better U.S. health care', Commonwealth Fund, July 2017, https://interactives.commonwealthfund.org/2017/july/mirror-mirror/

6 WHO, 'Patient safety', 13 September 2019, https://www.who.int/news-room/fact-sheets/detail/patient-safety

7 Leveson Inquiry, 'An inquiry into the culture, practices and ethics of the press: executive summary', Department for Digital, Culture, Media and Sport, 29 November 2012, https://assets.publishing.service.gov.uk/government/uploads/system/uploads/attachment_data/file/229039/0779.pdf

8 Patrick Wintour and Dan Sabbagh, 'Minister for Murdoch', *Guardian*, 25 April 2012.

9 Ruth Alexander, 'Which is the world's biggest employer?', BBC News, 20 March 2012, https://www.bbc.co.uk/news/magazine-17429786.

10 King's Fund, 'How the NHS is funded', 1 March 2021, https://www.kingsfund.org.uk/projects/nhs-in-a-nutshell/how-nhs-funded

11 BBC News, 'Cabinet reshuffle: Lansley replaced by Hunt in health job', 4 September 2012, https://www.bbc.co.uk/news/uk-politics-19472688

12 Francis Inquiry, 'Report of the Mid Staffordshire NHS Foundation Trust public inquiry', 6 February 2013, https://www.gov.uk/government/publications/report-of-the-mid-staffordshire-nhs-foundation-trust-public-inquiry

13 Helen Hogan et al., 'Avoidability of hospital deaths and association with hospital-wide mortality ratios: retrospective case record review and regression analysis', *BMJ*, 14 July 2015, p. 351.

14 CQC, 'Planning the inspection', https://www.cqc.org.uk/what-we-do/how-we-do-our-job/planning-inspection

15 CQC, 'The state of care in NHS acute hospitals: 2014 to 2016', 2 March 2017, https://www.cqc.org.uk/sites/default/files/20170302b_stateofhospitals_web.pdf

16 Full Fact, 'Are three million more patients using good or outstanding hospitals?', 9 July 2019, https://fullfact.org/health/three-million-more-patients-good-outstanding-hospitals/

17 Health and Social Care, and Science and Technology Committees, 'Coronavirus: lessons learned to date', 12 October 2021, https://publications.parliament.uk/pa/cm5802/cmselect/cmhealth/92/9203.htm

18 Bliss, 'Neonatal mortality in the UK', https://www.bliss.org.uk/research-campaigns/neonatal-care-statistics/neonatal-mortality-in-the-uk-how-many-babies-die-in-their-first-28-days-of-life

19 A. Zylbersztejn et al., 'Child mortality in England compared with Sweden: a birth cohort study', *Lancet* 391(10134), 2018, pp. 2008–18, https://www.ncbi.nlm.nih.gov/pmc/articles/PMC5958228/

Chapter 1: Blame

1 Kirkup Inquiry, 'The report of the Morecambe Bay investigation', March 2015, https://assets.publishing.service.gov.uk/government/uploads/system/uploads/attachment_data/file/408480/47487_MBI_Accessible_v0.1.pdf

2 BBC News, 'Liza Brady "devastated" after police drop baby death probe', 19 June 2013, https://www.bbc.co.uk/news/uk-england-22956240

3 Julie Mellor, 'Midwifery supervision and regulation: recommendations for change', Parliamentary and Health Service Ombudsman, December 2013. https://www.ombudsman.org.uk/publications/midwifery-supervision-and-regulation-recommendations-change/foreword-and-summary

4 Sara-Kate Templeton, 'Father's agony drives bid to cut stillbirths', *Sunday Times*, 3 December 2017, https://www.thetimes.co.uk/article/fathers-agony-drives-bid-to-cut-stillbirths-5qlf5bk0s

5 James Titcombe, *Joshua's Story: Uncovering the Morecambe Bay NHS Scandal* (Leeds: Anderson Wallace, 2015).

6 UK Sepsis Trust, 'The importance of asking: could it be sepsis?', https://sepsistrust.org/the-importance-of-asking-could-it-be-sepsis/

7 King's Fund, 'Activity in the NHS', 23 October 2020, https://www.kingsfund.org.uk/projects/nhs-in-a-nutshell/NHS-activity

8 James Titcombe, *Joshua's Story*, pp. 47 and 52.

9 Ibid., p. 121.

10 Albert W. Wu, 'Medical error: the second victim – the doctor who makes the mistake needs help too', *BMJ* 320(7237), 2000, pp. 726–27.

11 Julia Shaw, *The Memory Illusion: Remembering, Forgetting, and the Science of False Memory* (London: Random House, 2016).

12 Matthew Syed, *Black Box Thinking: The Surprising Truth About Success* (London: John Murray, 2015), pp. 22–33.

13 BBC News, '2017 safest year for air travel as fatalities fall', 2 January 2018, https://www.bbc.co.uk/news/business-42538053

14 Gwyn Topham, 'Ethiopian flight 302: second new Boeing 737 to crash in four months', *Guardian*, 10 March 2019, https://www.theguardian.com/world/2019/mar/10/ethiopian-flight-302-second-new-boeing-737-max-8-to-crash-in-four-months

15 US House Committee on Transportation and Infrastructure, 'Final committee report: the design, development and certification of the Boeing 737 Max', 2 September 2020, https://transportation.house.gov/download/20200915-final-737-max-report-for-public-release

16 David Marx, 'Patient safety and the "just culture": a primer for health care executives', Medical Event Reporting System for Transfusion Medicine/Columbia University, 17 April 2001, http://www.chpso.org/sites/main/files/file-attachments/marx_primer.pdf

17 Andy Burnham, Hansard HC vol 591 (21 January 2015), https://hansard.parliament.uk/Commons/2015-01-21/debates/15012193000001/NationalHealthService

18 Sophie Borland, 'Labour's cover-up on failing hospitals', *Daily Mail*, 3 October 2013, https://www.dailymail.co.uk/news/article-2443051/Labours-cover-failing-hospitals-Ministers-tried-silence-watchdog-eve-general-election.html; Isabel Oakeshott, 'Labour sues Hunt for "libel" tweet', *Sunday Times*, 6 October 2013, https://www.thetimes.co.uk/article/labour-sues-hunt-for-libel-tweet-0flpksf8swk; BBC News, 'Jeremy Hunt denies accusing Andy Burnham of NHS cover-up', 7 October 2013, https://www.bbc.co.uk/news/uk-politics-24434296

19 DHSC, 'Consultation outcome: statutory duty of candour for health and adult social care providers', 26 March 2014, https://www.gov.uk/government/consultations/statutory-duty-of-candour-for-health-and-adult-social-care-providers

20 CQC, 'University Hospitals of Morecambe Bay NHS Foundation Trust: quality report', 26 June 2014, https://api.cqc.org.uk/public/v1/reports/73214fbb-b737-4de3-934b-0cc09d814c0c?20210130233125

21 Ibid.

22 University Hospitals of Morecambe Bay NHS Foundation Trust, 'NHS Staff Survey results show higher than average morale and positive diversity scores at UHMBT', Latest News, 11 March 2021, https://www.uhmb.nhs.uk/news-and-events/latest-news/nhs-staff-survey-results-show-higher-average-morale-and-positive-diversity-scores-uhmbt

23 BBC News, 'Morecambe Bay NHS Foundation Trust back in "special measures"', 18 August 2021, https://www.bbc.co.uk/news/uk-england-cumbria-58258279

24 DHSC, 'Establishing the Healthcare Safety Investigation Branch', 12 May 2016 https://www.gov.uk/government/news/establishing-the-healthcare-safety-investigation-branch

25 See National Guardian, https://nationalguardian.org.uk

26 BBC News, 'Joshua Titcombe death: midwife suspended for nine months', 19 August 2016, https://www.bbc.co.uk/news/uk-england-cumbria-37128340

Chapter 2: Short-Staffing

1 ONS, 'International migration and the healthcare workforce', 15 August 2019, https://www.ons.gov.uk/peoplepopulationandcommunity/populationandmigration/internationalmigration/articles/internationalmigrationandthehealthcareworkforce/2019-08-15

2 Carl Baker, 'NHS staff from overseas: statistics', 20 September 2021, https://researchbriefings.files.parliament.uk/documents/CBP-7783/CBP-7783.pdf

3 WHO, 'Health workforce', https://www.who.int/health-topics/health-workforce#tab=tab_1

4 King's Fund, 'NHS hospital bed numbers: past, present, future', 5 November 2021, https://www.kingsfund.org.uk/publications/nhs-hospital-bed-numbers

5 BMA, 'BMA meeting: Doctors vote to limit number of medical students', 9 July 2008, https://www.bmj.com/content/337/bmj.a748

6 Francis Inquiry, 'Report'.

7 Julie Bailey, *From Ward to Whitehall: the Disaster at Mid Staffs Hospital* (Stafford: Cure The NHS, 2012).

8 Department of Health figures supplied to author when he was Health Secretary.

9 NHS Digital, 'NHS workforce statistics – September 2021 (including selected provisional statistics for October 2021)', 6 January 2022, https://digital.nhs.uk/data-and-information/publications/statistical/nhs-workforce-statistics/september-2021

10 Helen Whately, answer to written question from Jonathan Ashworth, 'Hospitals: staff – question for Department of Health and Social Care', UK Parliament Written Questions, Answers and Statements, 23 July 2020, https://questions-statements.parliament.uk/written-questions/detail/2020-07-08/71059

11 OECD, 'Number of medical doctors and nurses', Data Insights, 23 August 2021, https://www.oecd.org/coronavirus/en/data-insights/number-of-medical-doctors-and-nurses

12 WHO, 'Burn-out an "occupational phenomenon": international classification of diseases', 28 May 2019, https://www.who.int/news/item/28-05-2019-burn-out-an-occupational-phenomenon-international-classification-of-diseases

13 NHS Employers, 'Supporting our NHS people experiencing stress', 6 January 2022, https://www.nhsemployers.org/articles/supporting-our-nhs-people-experiencing-stress

14 Jeremy Hunt, 'New deal for general practice', speech at the Nelson Medical Practice, 19 June 2015, https://www.gov.uk/government/speeches/new-deal-for-general-practice

15 Full Fact, 'GP numbers: up or down?', 13 May 2019, https://fullfact.org/health/gp-numbers-or-down/

16 DHSC, 'Mandate to Health Education England', April 2017 to March 2018, https://assets.publishing.service.gov.uk/government/uploads/system/uploads/attachment_data/file/781806/Withdrawn_-_DHSC_mandate_to_Health_Education_England_-_April_2017_to_March_2018.pdf

17 Nick Triggle, 'Student doctor numbers to rise by 25%', BBC News, 4 October 2016, https://www.bbc.co.uk/news/health-37546360

18 Paul Gallagher, 'Jeremy Hunt announces an extra 5,000 nurse degree places', *i*, 3 October 2017, https://inews.co.uk/news/health/jeremy-hunt-plans-increase-nurse-degree-training-places-94873

19 Politics, 'Hunt NHS workforce amendment defeated', 23 November 2021, https://www.politics.co.uk/news-in-brief/hunt-nhs-workforce-amendment-defeated/

20 NHS Digital, 'NHS vacancy statistics England April 2015–September 2021', 25 November 2021, https://digital.nhs.uk/data-and-information/publications/statistical/nhs-vacancies-survey/april-2015---september-2021-experimental-statistics

21 Figures provided by various Royal Colleges.

Chapter 3: Money

1 NHS England, Cancer Drugs Fund, https://www.england.nhs.uk/cancer/cdf/

2 NHS England, 'NHS increases budget for cancer drugs fund from £280 million in 2014/15 to an expected £340 million in 2015/16', 12 January 2015, https://www.england.nhs.uk/2015/01/cancer-drug-budget/

3 OECD, 'Health spending (2020 or latest available)', https://data.oecd.org/healthres/health-spending.htm

4 Commonwealth Fund, 'Mirror, mirror 2021: reflecting poorly – health care in the U.S. compared to other high-income countries', 4 August 2021, https://www.commonwealthfund.org/publications/fund-reports/2021/aug/mirror-mirror-2021-reflecting-poorly#rank

5 ONS, 'National life tables – life expectancy in the UK: 2018 to 2020', 23 September 2021, https://www.ons.gov.uk/peoplepopulationandcommunity/birthsdeathsandmarriages/lifeexpectancies/bulletins/nationallifetablesunitedkingdom/2018to2020

6 Health Foundation, 'Understanding the health care needs of people with multiple health conditions', November 2018, citing Andrew Kingston et al., 'Projections of multi-morbidity in the older population in England to 2035: estimates from the Population Ageing and Care

Simulation (PACSim) model', *Age and Ageing* 47(3), May 2018, pp. 374–80, https://pubmed.ncbi.nlm.nih.gov/29370339/

7   King's Fund, 'Long-term conditions and multi-morbidity', https://www. kingsfund.org.uk/projects/time-think-differently/trends-disease-and-disability-long-term-conditions-multi-morbidity

8   James Gallagher, 'G8 "will develop dementia cure or treatment by 2025"', BBC News, 11 December 2013, https://www.bbc.co.uk/news/health-25318194

9   Resolution Foundation, 'The Boris budget', October 2021, https://www. resolutionfoundation.org/app/uploads/2021/10/The-Boris-Budget. pdf

10 NHS England, 'Five Year Forward View', October 2014, https://www. england.nhs.uk/wp-content/uploads/2014/10/5yfv-web.pdf

11 Nick Triggle, 'We want our Brexit cash boost – NHS boss', BBC News, 8 November 2017, https://www.bbc.co.uk/news/health-41908302

12 DHSC and HM Treasury, 'Prime Minister sets out 5-year NHS funding plan', 19 June 2018, https://www.gov.uk/government/news/prime-minister-sets-out-5-year-nhs-funding-plan

13 Data supplied by the DHSC to the author when he was Health Secretary.

14 Kevin Fenton, 'The human cost of falls', UK Health Security Agency, 17 July 2014, https://ukhsa.blog.gov.uk/2014/07/17/the-human-cost-of-falls/

15 Sherwood Forest Hospitals NHS Foundation Trust, 'Falls policy – prevention of patient falls', 30 December 2019, https://www.sfh-tr. nhs.uk/media/8918/falls-policy-prevention-of-patient-falls.pdf

16 NICE, 'Healthcare-associated infections: prevention and control in primary and community care – clinical guideline [CG139]', 15 February 2017, https://www.nice.org.uk/guidance/cg139/chapter/ introduction

17 Rachel Ann Elliott et al., 'Economic analysis of the prevalence and clinical and economic burden of medication error in England', *BMJ Quality & Safety* 2(30), February 2021 (epub June 2020), pp. 96–105.

18 Calculations worked out using the BMA's 'Pay scales for consultants in England' at https://www.bma.org.uk/pay-and-contracts/pay/

consultants-pay-scales/pay-scales-for-consultants-in-england, and the average cost of a nurse according to the Royal College of Nursing at https://www.nurses.co.uk/careers-hub/nursing-pay-guide/#average-wage-for-a-UK-Nurse-in-2021

19 Jeremy Hunt, 'How can we afford the kind of care we all want?', article, 2 June 2015, https://www.gov.uk/government/speeches/how-can-we-afford-the-kind-of-care-we-all-want

Chapter 4: Targets

1 Francis Inquiry, 'Report'.
2 Overall summary of this period provided by the King's Fund, see 'How much has been spent on the NHS since 2005?', https://www.kingsfund.org.uk/projects/general-election-2010/money-spent-nhs and 'How much have waiting times reduced?', https://www.kingsfund.org.uk/projects/general-election-2010/waiting-times
3 Health Foundation, 'Infection prevention and control: lessons from acute care in England', November 2015, https://www.health.org.uk/sites/default/files/InfectionPreventionAndControlLessonsFromAcute CareInEngland.pdf, p. 8 for MRSA and p. 9 for C. diff.
4 Francis Inquiry, 'Report'.
5 See Cure the NHS, http://www.curethenhs.co.uk
6 Francis Inquiry, 'Report of the Mid Staffordshire inquiry: executive summary', https://assets.publishing.service.gov.uk/government/uploads/system/uploads/attachment_data/file/279124/0947.pdf
7 Health Committee, 'Minutes of evidence', 17 September 2013, https://publications.parliament.uk/pa/cm201314/cmselect/cmhealth/657/130305.htm
8 Examples include the following media reports at the time: Eve McQuillan, 'I've been waiting so long for an operation on the NHS that I could lose the use of my hand forever', *Independent*, 11 August 2017, https://www.independent.co.uk/voices/nhs-operation-waiting-times-too-long-cuts-healthcare-jeremy-hunt-conservative-government-a7887756.html and Nick McDermott, 'Crisis point:

Jeremy Hunt admits the NHS has suffered its "worst ever" winter amid record A & E wait times', *Sun*, 8 February 2013, https://www.thesun.co.uk/news/5532553/jeremy-hunt-admits-the-nhs-has-suffered-its-worst-ever-winter-amid-record-ae-wait-times/

9 King's Fund, 'How much have waiting times reduced?'

10 Public Health England, 'MRSA, MSSA and Gram-negative bacteraemia and CDI: annual report', 15 September 2021, https://www.gov.uk/government/statistics/mrsa-mssa-and-e-coli-bacteraemia-and-c-difficile-infection-annual-epidemiological-commentary

11 NHS, 'Guide to NHS waiting times in England', 2 December 2019, https://www.nhs.uk/nhs-services/hospitals/guide-to-nhs-waiting-times-in-england/

12 Alex Bate, Carl Baker and Andrew Mackley, 'NHS cancer targets', research briefing, 30 April 2018, https://researchbriefings.files.parliament.uk/documents/CDP-2018-0105/CDP-2018-0105.pdf

13 NHS, 'NHS England proposes new mental health access standards', 22 July 2021, https://www.england.nhs.uk/2021/07/nhs-england-proposes-new-mental-health-access-standards/

14 Public Health England, 'Gram-negative bacteria: prevention, surveillance and epidemiology', 1 August 2017, https://www.gov.uk/guidance/gram-negative-bacteria-prevention-surveillance-and-epidemiology

15 NHS England, DHSC and Public Health England, 'The national flu immunisations programme 2020 to 2021', letter, 5 August 2020, https://www.england.nhs.uk/wp-content/uploads/2020/05/Letter_AnnualFlu_2020-21_20200805.pdf

16 DHSC, 'New ambition to halve rate of stillbirths and infant deaths', 13 November 2015, https://www.gov.uk/government/news/new-ambition-to-halve-rate-of-stillbirths-and-infant-deaths

17 DHSC, 'Health Secretary announces goal to end HIV transmissions by 2030', 30 January 2019, https://www.gov.uk/government/news/health-secretary-announces-goal-to-end-hiv-transmissions-by-2030

18 DHSC, 'New ambition to halve rate of stillbirths and infant deaths'.

19 NHS England, 'New plans to improve dementia diagnosis rates', 15 May 2013, https://www.england.nhs.uk/2013/05/dementia-targets

20 DHSC, 'Reducing infections in the NHS', 20 December 2016, https://www.gov.uk/government/news/reducing-infections-in-the-nhs

21 DHSC, 'Government strengthens health regulator's independence', 1 October 2013, https://www.gov.uk/government/news/government-strengthens-health-regulators-independence

22 Full Fact, 'Are three million more patients using good or outstanding hospitals?' It was nearly three million more additional patients whilst the author was in office but has now risen to four million.

23 CQC, 'Routine inspections suspended in response to coronavirus outbreak', 16 March 2020, https://www.cqc.org.uk/news/stories/routine-inspections-suspended-response-coronavirus-outbreak

24 DHSC, 'Government launches NHS Test and Trace service', 27 May 2020, https://www.gov.uk/government/news/government-launches-nhs-test-and-trace-service

25 DHSC, 'Health Secretary sets out plan to carry out 100,000 coronavirus tests a day', 2 April 2020, https://www.gov.uk/government/news/health-secretary-sets-out-plan-to-carry-out-100000-coronavirus-tests-a-day

26 Charles Goodhart, 'Problems of monetary management: the U.K. experience', *Papers in Monetary Economics, Volume 1* (Sydney: Reserve Bank of Australia, 1975).

27 Full Fact, 'Did the government meet its Covid-19 test targets?', 10 July 2020, https://fullfact.org/health/six-test-targets/

28 Health and Social Care, and Science and Technology Committees, 'Coronavirus: lessons learned to date', 21 September 2021, https://committees.parliament.uk/publications/7496/documents/78687/default/, p. 77.

29 King's Fund, 'NHS waiting lists: how big is big?', 11 November 2021, https://www.kingsfund.org.uk/blog/2021/11/nhs-waiting-lists-how-big

30 HMRC, 'Health and social care levy', 13 December 2021, https://www.gov.uk/government/publications/health-and-social-care-levy/health-and-social-care-levy

Chapter 5: Hierarchies

1   EMCrit, 'The case of Elaine Bromiley', https://emcrit.org/wp-content/uploads/ElaineBromileyAnonymousReport.pdf

2   Husam Kharoufah et al., 'A review of human factors causations in commercial air transport accidents and incidents: from to 2000–2016', *Progress in Aerospace Sciences* 99, May 2018, pp. 1–13.

3   See https://chfg.org

4   World Bank, 'Air transport, passengers carried', https://data.worldbank.org/indicator/IS.AIR.PSGR

5   Aviation Safety Network, 'Statistics by period', https://aviation-safety.net/statistics/period/stats.php

6   Francis Inquiry, 'Report of the Mid Staffordshire NHS Foundation Trust public inquiry – Volume 1: Analysis of evidence and lessons learned (part 1)', 6 February 2013, https://assets.publishing.service.gov.uk/government/uploads/system/uploads/attachment_data/file/279115/0898_i.pdf

7   Socialist Health Association, 'Griffiths Report on NHS October 1983', 6 October 1983, https://www.sochealth.co.uk/national-health-service/griffiths-report-october-1983/

8   Jim Collins, *Good To Great: Why Some Companies Make the Leap... and Others Don't* (London: Random House Business, 2001).

9   Jerry Large, 'Tragic death drives quest for patient safety at Seattle hospital', *Seattle Times*, 12 June 2016, https://www.seattletimes.com/seattle-news/tragic-death-drives-quest-for-patient-safety-at-seattle-hospital/

10 For the US see Amir A. Khaliq and David M. Thompson, 'The impact of hospital CEO turnover in U.S. hospitals: final report', 27 February 2006, https://citeseerx.ist.psu.edu/viewdoc/download?doi=10.1.1.619.9124&rep=rep1&type=pdf; for the UK, see Siva Anandaciva et al., 'Leadership in today's NHS: delivering the impossible', King's Fund, July 2018, https://www.kingsfund.org.uk/sites/default/files/2018-07/Leadership_in_todays_NHS.pdf

11 Virginia Mason Franciscan Health, 'Virginia Mason ranks among best

hospitals in U.S. News & World Report annual survey', 28 July 2020, https://www.virginiamason.org/virginia-mason-ranks-among-best-hospitals-in-u-s-news-world-report-annual-survey

12 Western Sussex Hospitals NHS Foundation Trust, 'CQC rating: outstanding', 22 October 2019, https://www.westernsussexhospitals.nhs.uk/your-trust/performance/cqc-rating-outstanding/

13 University Hospitals Sussex NHS Foundation Trust, 'Dame Marianne Griffiths announces retirement', 14 October 2021, https://www.uhsussex.nhs.uk/dame-marianne-griffiths-announces-retirement/

14 Victor Davis Hanson, *Carnage and Culture: Landmark Battles in the Rise to Western Power* (London: Bantam Dell, 2002).

Chapter 6: Litigation

1 Clare Dyer, 'Doctors suspended after injecting wrong drug into spine', *BMJ*, 3 February 2001, https://www.bmj.com/content/322/7281/257.1.extract

2 For the GMC's summary, see GMC, 'Responding to the case of Dr Bawa-Garba', https://www.gmc-uk.org/about/how-we-work/corporate-strategy-plans-and-impact/supporting-a-profession-under-pressure/responding-to-the-case-of-dr-bawa-garba

3 Court of Appeal (Civil Division), *Bawa-Garba v. GMC*, Approved Judgement, 13 October 2018, https://www.judiciary.uk/wp-content/uploads/2018/08/bawa-garba-v-gmc-final-judgment-1.pdf

4 BBC News, 'Jeremy Hunt says doctors must be allowed to discuss mistakes', 26 January 2018, https://www.bbc.co.uk/news/health-42833028

5 BBC News, 'Jack Adcock manslaughter: convicted doctor "fit to practise"', 2 July 2021, https://www.bbc.co.uk/news/uk-england-leicestershire-57700681

6 BBC News, 'Hunt orders review of criminalising doctors after Bawa-Garba case', 6 February 2018, https://www.bbc.co.uk/news/health-42958391

7 NHS Resolution, 'Annual report and accounts 2020/21', https:// resolution.nhs.uk/wp-content/uploads/2021/07/Annual-report-and-accounts-2020-21-web.pdf#page=42

8 Shaun Lintern, 'Family wins £37m in one of the largest maternity negligence claims in NHS history', *Independent*, 20 July 2020, https://www.independent.co.uk/news/health/maternity-safety-nhs-negligence-guys-thomas-a9357501.html

9 £600 million is paid in fees to lawyers. Calculation based on Royal College of Nursing average salary information and BMA consultant pay scales (op. cit.).

10 Operating costs are £1.9 billion compared to £2.3 billion in compensation costs. See Barts Health NHS Trust, 'Annual reports and accounts 2020–2021', https://www.bartshealth.nhs.uk/download. cfm?doc=docm93jijm4n19009.pdf&ver=34511

11 NHS Resolution, 'Annual reports and accounts 2020/21'.

12 Helen Whately, answer to written question from Jeremy Hunt, 'Maternity services: pay', UK Parliament Written Questions, Answers and Statements, 11 June 2020, https://questions-statements.parliament. uk/written-questions/detail/2020-05-18/48342/

13 Health and Social Care Committee, 'The safety of maternity services in England', 6 July 2021, https://publications.parliament.uk/pa/cm5802/ cmselect/cmhealth/19/1904.htm

14 Statista, 'Number of stillborn children in Sweden from 2010 to 2020 (per 1,000 births)', 2 February 2022, https://www.statista.com/ statistics/524771/sweden-infant-mortality-rate/

15 World Bank, 'Mortality rate, neonatal (per 1,000 live births) – Sweden (2020)', https://data.worldbank.org/indicator/SH.DYN. NMRT?locations=SE

16 ONS, 'Vital statistics in the UK: births, deaths and marriages (2020)', 3 December 2021, https://www.ons.gov.uk/peoplepopulationand community/populationandmigration/populationestimates/datasets/ vitalstatisticspopulationandhealthreferencetables

17 Socialstyrelsen, 'Statistics on pregnancies, deliveries and newborn infants 2020', 1 December 2021, https://www.socialstyrelsen.se/

globalassets/sharepoint-dokument/artikelkatalog/statistik/2021-12-7653.pdf

18 NHS Digital, 'NHS maternity statistics, England 2019–20', 29 October 2020, https://digital.nhs.uk/data-and-information/publications/statistical/nhs-maternity-statistics/2019-20#resources

19 NHS Digital, 'Maternity services monthly statistics (2020)', https://digital.nhs.uk/data-and-information/publications/statistical/maternity-services-monthly-statistics

20 More information on the scheme can be found at Löf, https://lof.se/language/engelska-english

21 Health and Social Care Committee, 'Supplementary written evidence submitted by the Department of Health and Social Care (NLR 0072)', January 2022, https://committees.parliament.uk/writtenevidence/42609/pdf/

22 Health and Social Care Committee, 'Oral evidence: NHS litigation reform', 11 January 2022, https://committees.parliament.uk/oralevidence/3255/html/

23 ONS, 'Child and infant mortality in England and Wales 2020', 17 February 2022, https://www.ons.gov.uk/peoplepopulationandcommunity/birthsdeathsandmarriages/deaths/bulletins/childhoodinfantand perinatalmortalityinenglandandwales/2020

24 DHSC, 'Improving the safety of maternity care in the NHS', 17 October 2016, https://www.gov.uk/government/news/improving-the-safety-of-maternity-care-in-the-nhs

25 See Healthcare Safety and Investigation Branch, https://www.hsib.org.uk/

26 Professor Sir Norman Williams Review report, 11 June 2018, https://www.gov.uk/government/groups/professor-sir-norman-williams-review

Chapter 7: Groupthink

1 For the latest data, see ONS, 'Influenza deaths in 2018, 2019 and 2020', 24 February 2021, https://www.ons.gov.uk/aboutus/

transparencyandgovernance/freedomofinformationfoi/influenzade athsin20182019and2020

2 DHSC, 'Annex B: Exercise Cygnus Report', 5 November 2020, https://www.gov.uk/government/publications/uk-pandemic-preparedness/exercise-cygnus-report-accessible-report

3 Coronavirus Act 2020, https://www.legislation.gov.uk/ukpga/2020/7/contents/enacted

4 World Economic Forum, 'These are the countries best prepared for health emergencies', 12 February 2020, https://www.weforum.org/agenda/2020/02/these-are-the-countries-best-prepared-for-health-emergencies/

5 Greta Privitera, 'Italian doctors on coronavirus frontline face tough calls on whom to save', *Politico*, 9 March 2020, https://www.politico.eu/article/coronavirus-italy-doctors-tough-calls-survival/

6 Simiao Chen et al., 'Fangcang shelter hospitals: a novel concept for responding to public health emergencies', *Lancet* 395(10232), 18–24 April 2020, pp. 1305–14, https://www.ncbi.nlm.nih.gov/pmc/articles/PMC7270591/

7 NHS England, 'NHS steps up coronavirus fight with two more Nightingale Hospitals', 10 April 2020, https://www.england.nhs.uk/2020/04/nhs-steps-up-coronavirus-fight-with-two-more-nightingale-hospitals/

8 Lucy Fisher, 'It's my biggest mission, says colonel who built Nightingale Hospital', *The Times*, 1 April 2020, https://www.thetimes.co.uk/article/its-my-biggest-mission-says-colonel-who-built-nightingale-hospital-wmp6ckvhx

9 Cancer Research UK, 'One year on: how has COVID-19 affected cancer services?' 14 May 2021, https://news.cancerresearchuk.org/2021/05/14/one-year-on-how-has-covid-19-affected-cancer-services/

10 NHS estimate provided to the Health and Social Care Committee, 'Oral evidence: Cancer Services', 20 January 2022, https://committees.parliament.uk/oralevidence/3317/html/

11 BBC News, 'Covid-19 vaccine: First person receives Pfizer jab in UK', 8 December 2020, https://www.bbc.co.uk/news/uk-55227325

12 British Embassy Beijing and British Consulates General Guangzhou, Chongqing, Shanghai and Wuhan, 'UK takes drastic measures to tackle COVID-19', 18 March 2020, https://www.gov.uk/government/news/uk-takes-drastic-measures-to-tackle-covid-19

13 Widely reported at the time, see e.g. Steerpike, 'Five howlers from Jenny Harries', *Spectator*, 28 December 2021, https://www.spectator.co.uk/article/five-howlers-of-jenny-harries

14 Hannah Ritchie et al., 'South Korea: coronavirus pandemic country profile', 2020, Our World In Data, https://ourworldindata.org/coronavirus/country/south-korea

15 ONS, 'International comparisons of GDP during the coronavirus (COVID-19) pandemic', 1 February 2021, https://www.ons.gov.uk/economy/gross domesticproductgdp/articles/internationalcomparisonsofgdpduringthe coronaviruscovid19pandemic/2021-02-01

16 Rajiv Biswas, 'South Korea economic rebound threatened by new COVID wave', IHS Markit, 2 August 2021, citing Bank of Korea data for 2020, https://ihsmarkit.com/research-analysis/south-korea-economic-rebound-threatened-by-new-covid-wave-Aug21.html

17 Health and Social Care, and Science and Technology Committees, 'Coronavirus: lessons learned to date', 21 September 2021', https://committees.parliament.uk/publications/7496/documents/78687/default/

18 As reported in Nina Strochlic and Riley D. Champine, 'How some cities "flattened the curve" during the 1918 flu pandemic', *National Geographic*, 27 March 2020, https://www.nationalgeographic.com/history/article/how-cities-flattened-curve-1918-spanish-flu-pandemic-coronavirus

19 Sergio Correia, Stephan Luck and Emil Verner, 'Pandemics depress the economy, public health interventions do not: evidence from the 1918 flu', *SSRN*, 5 June 2020, http://dx.doi.org/10.2139/ssrn.3561560

20 Ibid.

21 Health and Social Care, and Science and Technology Committees, 'Oral evidence: coronavirus: lessons learnt', 10 June 2021, https://committees.parliament.uk/oralevidence/2318/html/

22 Idem, 'Oral evidence: coronavirus: lessons learnt', 26 May 2021, https://committees.parliament.uk/oralevidence/2249/html/

23 Public Health England, 'Report: Exercise Alice Middle East Respiratory Syndrome Coronavirus (MERS-CoV', 15 February 2016, https://cygnusreports.org/wp-content/uploads/2021/10/Report-Exercise-Alice-Middle-East-Respiratory-Syndrome-15-Feb-2016.pdf

24 ONS, 'Rolling annual death registrations by place of occurrence', 4 June 2020, https://www.ons.gov.uk/peoplepopulationandcommunity/birthsdeathsandmarriages/deaths/adhocs/11820rollingannualdeathregistrationsbyplaceofoccurrenceenglandperiodendingquarter4jantomaroffinancialyear2019to2020. This shows that 223,000 of the 500,000 deaths in 2019–20 occurred in hospital in 191 Clinical Commissioning Groups, with an average of 1,170 in each.

25 Helen Hogan et al., 'Avoidability of hospital deaths', p. 351.

26 BBC News, 'Li Wenliang: Coronavirus kills Chinese whistleblower doctor', 7 February 2020, https://www.bbc.co.uk/news/world-asia-china-51403795

27 'Obituary: Li Wenliang', Economist, 15 February 2020, https://www.economist.com/obituary/2020/02/13/li-wenliang-died-on-february-7th

28 BBC News, 'Li Wenliang'.

29 University of Southampton, 'Early and combined interventions crucial in tackling Covid-19 spread in China', 11 March 2020, https://www.southampton.ac.uk/news/2020/03/covid-19-china.page

Chapter 8: Transparency

1 See NHS England, 'Professor Tim Kendall', https://www.england.nhs.uk/author/professor-tim-kendall/

2 NBC News, 'Clinton: being president like being cemetery superintendent', 25 February 2014, https://www.nbcnews.com/video/clinton-being-president-like-being-cemetery-superintendent-170020931651

3 Data supplied by Tim Briggs.

4 See for instance Sheffield Teaching Hospitals NHS Foundation Trust, 'Osteoporosis drug could half number of redo hip replacement

operations', 12 January 2021, https://www.sth.nhs.uk/news/news?action=view&newsID=1275

5   Tim Briggs, 'Getting it right in orthopaedics: reflecting on success and reinforcing improvement', GIRFT, February 2022, https://gettingitrightfirsttime.co.uk/wp-content/uploads/2020/02/GIRFT-orthopaedics-follow-up-report-February-2020.pdf, p. 62

6   Ibid.

7   GIRFT, 'Litigation', https://www.gettingitrightfirsttime.co.uk/cross-cutting-stream/litigation/

8   GIRFT, 'What we do', https://www.gettingitrightfirsttime.co.uk/what-we-do/

9   Queensland Government, 'Getting it Right First Time', https://clinicalexcellence.qld.gov.au/priority-areas/service-improvement/girft

10   GIRFT, 'NCIP', https://www.gettingitrightfirsttime.co.uk/ncip

11   DHSC, 'New maternity strategy to reduce the number of stillbirths', 28 November 2017, https://www.gov.uk/government/news/new-maternity-strategy-to-reduce-the-number-of-stillbirths; and see ONS, 'Child and infant mortality in England and Wales 2020'.

12   Health and Social Care Committee, 'The Health and Social Care Committee's expert panel: evaluation of the government's progress against its policy commitments in the area of maternity services in England – first special report', 30 June 2021, https://committees.parliament.uk/publications/6560/documents/71747/default/

13   Royal College of Surgeons of England, 'Prof Norman Williams President on publication of surgeon level outcome data', 13 June 2013, https://www.rcseng.ac.uk/news-and-events/media-centre/press-releases/publication-of-surgeon-level-outcome-data/

14   Laura Donnelly, 'NHS surgeons with the highest death rates named', *Daily Telegraph*, 28 June 2013, https://www.telegraph.co.uk/news/politics/10147355/NHS-surgeons-with-the-highest-death-rates-named.html

15   Samer Nashef, *The Naked Surgeon: The Power and Peril of Transparency in Medicine* (London: Scribe, 2015).

16 Nadine Dorries, answer to written question from Jeremy Hunt, 'NHS trusts: standards – question for Department of Health and Social Care', UK Parliament Written Questions, Answers and Statements, 11 May 2020, https://questions-statements.parliament.uk/written-questions/detail/2020-05-04/42952

Chapter 9: Continuity

1 Larisa Brown, 'Our health heroes', *Daily Mail*, 13 June 2013, https://www.dailymail.co.uk/news/article-2341339/Our-health-heroes-Devoted-GP-visited-dying-patient-hours-leads-line-unsung-stars-NHS.html

2 Natalie Clarke and India Sturgis, 'Meet the *Mail*'s health heroes', *Daily Mail*, 18 June 2013, https://www.dailymail.co.uk/health/article-2343408/Meet-Mail-Health-Heroes-From-GP-whos-ALWAYS-surgeon-sings-comfort-scared-children-extra-mile.html

3 Hogne Sandvik et al., 'Continuity in general practice as predictor of mortality, acute hospitalisation, and use of out-of-hours care: a registry-based observational study in Norway', *British Journal of General Practice* 72(715), 2022 (epub 2021), pp. e84–90.

4 Denis J. Pereira Gray et al., 'Continuity of care with doctors – a matter of life and death? A systematic review of continuity of care and mortality', *BMJ Open* 8(6), June 2018; Richard Baker, 'Primary medical care continuity and patient mortality: a systematic review', *British Journal of General Practice* 70(698), 2020, pp. e600–11.

5 NHS England, 'GP patient survey 2019', 11 July 2019, https://www.england.nhs.uk/statistics/2019/07/11/gp-patient-survey-2019

6 DHSC, 'Personalised GP care for everyone', 30 September 2014, https://www.gov.uk/government/news/personalised-gp-care-for-everyone

7 Monitor, 'Implementing the "responsible consultant/clinician" and "named nurse" in your NHS foundation trust', 24 October 2014, https://www.gov.uk/government/publications/implementing-the-responsible-consultantclinician-and-named-nurse-in-your-nhs-foundation-trust

8 OECD, 'Life expectancy at birth (2020 or latest available)', https://data.oecd.org/healthstat/life-expectancy-at-birth.htm

9 WHO, 'Healthy life expectancy (HALE) at birth (years)', 4 December 2020, https://www.who.int/data/gho/data/indicators/indicator-details/GHO/gho-ghe-hale-healthy-life-expectancy-at-birth

10 Health and Social Care Committee, 'Oral evidence: management of the coronavirus outbreak', 9 June 2020, https://committees.parliament.uk/oralevidence/482/html/

11 Tim Briggs, 'Getting it right in orthopaedics', p. 27.

12 Carehome.co.uk, 'Care home fees and costs: how much do you pay?', September 2021, https://www.carehome.co.uk/advice/care-home-fees-and-costs-how-much-do-you-pay

13 UK Care Guide, 'How much does in home care cost in 2022', 1 February 2022, https://ukcareguide.co.uk/home-care-costs/

14 See Surrey and Borders Partnership NHS Foundation Trust, 'TIHM monitoring service', https://www.sabp.nhs.uk/tihm/about

15 NHS Digital, 'Payment by results', 21 January 2019, https://digital.nhs.uk/data-and-information/data-tools-and-services/data-services/hospital-episode-statistics/payment-by-results

16 See Nuffield Trust, 'What can England learn from the long-term care system in Germany?', 11 September 2019, https://www.nuffieldtrust.org.uk/research/what-can-england-learn-from-the-long-term-care-system-in-germany, and 'What can England learn from the long-term care system in Japan?', 9 May 2018, https://www.nuffieldtrust.org.uk/research/what-can-england-learn-from-the-long-term-care-system-in-japan

Chapter 10: Homecare

1 My Daft Life, https://mydaftlife.com

2 Sara Ryan, *Justice for Laughing Boy: Connor Sparrowhawk – A Death by Indifference* (London: Jessica Kingsley Publishers, 2017).

3 Katrina Percy, 'A day in the life of a foundation trust chief executive', *Guardian*, 8 February 2013, https://www.theguardian.com/healthcare-network/2013/feb/08/foundation-trust-chief-executive-day-life

4 NHS England, 'Independent review of deaths of people with a learning disability or mental health problem in contact with Southern Health NHS Foundation Trust April 2011 to March 2015', 16 December 2015, https://www.england.nhs.uk/south/wp-content/uploads/sites/6/2015/12/mazars-rep.pdf

5 BBC News, 'Southern Health fined £2m over deaths of two patients', 26 March 2018, https://www.bbc.co.uk/news/uk-england-43542284

6 Public Health England, 'People with learning disabilities had higher death rate from COVID-19', 12 November 2020, https://www.gov.uk/government/news/people-with-learning-disabilities-had-higher-death-rate-from-covid-19

7 Rotherham, Doncaster and South Humber NHS Foundation Trust and Niche Health and Social Care Consulting, 'Learning lessons – the care and treatment of Annette', July 2020, https://oesn11hpbml2xaq003wx02ib-wpengine.netdna-ssl.com/wp-content/uploads/2020/10/Public-Board-of-Directors-23-October-2020-v3.pdf

8 Health and Social Care Committee, 'The treatment of autistic people and people with learning disabilities: fifth report', 6 July 2021, https://committees.parliament.uk/publications/6669/documents/71689/default/

9 Ibid.

10 'Undercover care: abuse exposed', *Panorama*, 31 May 2011, https://www.bbc.co.uk/programmes/b011pwt6

11 BBC News, 'Winterbourne View: care workers jailed for abuse', 26 October 2012, https://www.bbc.co.uk/news/uk-england-bristol-20092894

12 BBC News, 'Arden Vale becomes third Castlebeck care home to close', 17 August 2011, https://www.bbc.co.uk/news/uk-england-birmingham-14563038

13 BBC News, 'Yew Trees hospital: Police confirm "abuse" investigation', 24 September 2020, https://www.bbc.co.uk/news/uk-england-essex-54280560

14 Health and Social Care Committee, 'The treatment of autistic people and people with learning disabilities'.

15 Tobias Jones, '*The Man Who Closed the Asylums: Franco Basaglia and the Revolution in Mental Health Care* by John Foot – review', *Guardian*, 19 August 2015, https://www.theguardian.com/books/2015/aug/19/man-who-closed-asylums-franco-basaglia-review

16 King's Fund, 'Case study 1: deinstitutionalisation in UK mental health services', https://www.kingsfund.org.uk/publications/making-change-possible/mental-health-services

17 DHSC, 'NHS becomes first healthcare system in the world to publish numbers of avoidable deaths', 14 December 2017, https://www.gov.uk/government/news/nhs-becomes-first-healthcare-system-in-the-world-to-publish-numbers-of-avoidable-deaths

18 See NHS Health Education England, 'The Oliver McGowan Mandatory Training in Learning Disability and Autism', https://www.hee.nhs.uk/our-work/learning-disability/oliver-mcgowan-mandatory-training-learning-disability-autism

19 NHS England, 'Stopping over medication of people with a learning disability, autism or both (STOMP)', https://www.england.nhs.uk/learning-disabilities/improving-health/stomp/

20 Mencap, 'Eight in 10 deaths of people with a learning disability are COVID related as inequality soars', 2 February 2021, https://www.mencap.org.uk/press-release/eight-10-deaths-people-learning-disability-are-covid-related-inequality-soars

Chapter 11: Prevention

1 NHS England, 'Root cause analysis investigation report 2014/41975', May 2016, https://www.england.nhs.uk/south/wp-content/uploads/sites/6/2015/03/root-cause-analysis-wm-report.pdf

2 WHO, 'Sepsis', 26 August 2020, https://www.who.int/news-room/fact-sheets/detail/sepsis

3 UK Sepsis Trust, https://sepsistrust.org

4 NHS, 'E-sepsis: early detection and treatment helping to save lives', https://www.longtermplan.nhs.uk/case-studies/esepsis/

5 NHS Digital, 'Prescriptions dispensed in the community – statistics

for England, 2007–2017', 28 June 2018, https://digital.nhs.uk/data-and-information/publications/statistical/prescriptions-dispensed-in-the-community/prescriptions-dispensed-in-the-community-england---2007---2017

6 'Thalidomide scandal: 60-year timeline', *Guardian*, 1 September 2012, https://www.theguardian.com/society/2012/sep/01/thalidomide-scandal-timeline

7 DHSC, 'Independent medicines and medical devices safety review report', 8 July 2020, https://www.gov.uk/government/publications/independent-medicines-and-medical-devices-safety-review-report

8 Policy Research Unit in Economic Evaluation of Health and Care Interventions, 'Prevalence and economic burden of medication errors in the NHS in England', 22 February 2018, http://www.eepru.org.uk/wp-content/uploads/2020/03/medication-error-report-edited-27032020.pdf

9 Danielle Ofri, *When We Do Harm: A Doctor Confronts Medical Error* (Boston, MA: Beacon Press, 2021).

10 Erin P. Balogh, Bryan T. Miller and John R. Ball, eds, *Improving Diagnosis in Health Care* (Washington, DC: National Academies Press, 2015).

11 Alexander Hodkinson et al., 'Preventable medication harm across health care settings: a systematic review and meta-analysis', *BMC Medicine* 18, 2020, https://doi.org/10.1186/s12916-020-01774-9

12 WHO, 'Medication without harm', https://www.who.int/initiatives/medication-without-harm

13 Elena Myasoedova et al., 'Increased incidence and impact of upper and lower gastrointestinal events in patients with rheumatoid arthritis in Olmsted County, Minnesota: a longitudinal population-based study', *Journal of Rheumatology* 39(7), July 2012, pp. 1355–62, https://www.ncbi.nlm.nih.gov/pmc/articles/PMC3389143/

14 DHSC, 'New funding to help hospitals introduce digital prescribing', 17 September 2020, https://www.gov.uk/government/news/new-funding-to-help-hospitals-introduce-digital-prescribing

15 'GPs have almost twice the safe number of patient contacts a day', *Pulse*, 18 January 2018, https://www.pulsetoday.co.uk/news/workforce/gps-have-almost-twice-the-safe-number-of-patient-contacts-a-day/

Chapter 12: Technology

1 Tim Worstall, 'Apparently the NHS is the world's largest buyer of fax machines', Adam Smith Institute, 13 July 2018, https://www.adamsmith.org/blog/apparently-the-nhs-is-the-worlds-largest-buyer-of-fax-machines. For the US, see Lloyd Minor, 'Why your doctor's office still depends on a fax machine', *Wall Street Journal*, 19 September 2019, https://www.wsj.com/articles/why-your-doctors-office-still-depends-on-a-fax-machine-01568918733 and Sarah Kliff and Margot Sanger-Katz, 'Bottleneck for U.S. coronavirus response: the fax machine', *New York Times*, 13 July 2020, https://www.nytimes.com/2020/07/13/upshot/coronavirus-response-fax-machines.html; for Germany, see Sabine Kinkartz, 'German health care: tackling COVID with paper, pen and a fax machine', *DW*, 27 January 2021, https://www.dw.com/en/german-health-care-tackling-covid-with-paper-pen-and-a-fax-machine/a-56360491

2 DHSC, 'Health and Social Care Secretary bans fax machines in NHS', 9 December 2018, https://www.gov.uk/government/news/health-and-social-care-secretary-bans-fax-machines-in-nhs

3 NHS, 'Connecting for Health: a guide to the national programme for information technology', April 2005, https://web.archive.org/web/20051026213141/http://www.connectingforhealth.nhs.uk/all_images_and_docs/NPfIT%20brochure%20Apr%2005%20final.pdf

4 DHSC, 'Jeremy Hunt challenges NHS to go paperless by 2018', 16 January 2013, https://www.gov.uk/government/news/jeremy-hunt-challenges-nhs-to-go-paperless-by-2018

5 Robert M. Wachter, *The Digital Doctor: Hope, Hype, and Harm at the Dawn of Medicine's Computer Age* (New York: McGraw Hill, 2015).

6 See https://thriva.co/how-it-works

7 Eric Topol, *The Patient Will See You Now: The Future of Medicine is in Your Hands* (New York: Basic Books, 2015).

8 Emma Hill, 'Smart patients', *Lancet Oncology* 15(2), February 2014, pp. 140–1, https://www.thelancet.com/journals/lanonc/article/PIIS1470-2045(14)70044-0/fulltext?

9 Angelina Jolie, 'My medical choice', *New York Times*, 14 May 2013, https://www.nytimes.com/2013/05/14/opinion/my-medical-choice.html

Chapter 13: Communication

1 Jeremy Hunt, Hansard HC vol 605 (11 February 2016), https://hansard.parliament.uk/commons/2016-02-11/debates/16021153000002/JuniorDoctorsContracts

2 BBC News, 'Election 2015: Cameron promises "seven-day NHS" by 2020', 28 March 2015, https://www.bbc.co.uk/news/32094681

3 Nick Fremantle et al., 'Increased mortality associated with weekend hospital admission: a case for expanded seven day services?', *BMJ* 351, 5 September 2015, https://www.bmj.com/content/351/bmj.h4596

4 DHSC, 'Research into "the weekend effect" on patient outcomes and mortality', 30 October 2015, https://www.gov.uk/government/publications/research-into-the-weekend-effect-on-hospital-mortality/research-into-the-weekend-effect-on-patient-outcomes-and-mortality#aomrc-2012

5 Ibid.

6 King's Fund, 'Jeremy Hunt sets out his 25-year vision for the NHS', 16 July 2015, https://www.kingsfund.org.uk/audio-video/jeremy-hunt-sets-out-his-25-year-vision-nhs

7 Victoria Ward and Laura Donnelly, 'Jeremy Hunt goes to war with doctors – as it happened', 16 July 2015, https://www.telegraph.co.uk/news/nhs/11743103/Jeremy-Hunt-goes-to-war-with-doctors-as-it-happened.html

8 Nick Triggle, 'Junior doctors row: 98% vote in favour of strikes', BBC News, 19 November 2015, https://www.bbc.co.uk/news/health-34859860

9 Shaun Lintern, 'Exclusive: huge leak reveals BMA plan to "draw out" junior doctors dispute', *HSJ*, 26 May 2016, https://www.hsj.co.uk/workforce/exclusive-huge-leak-reveals-bma-plan-to-draw-out-junior-doctors-dispute/7005113.article?blocktitle=News&contentID=15303

10 NHS England, 'Never Events policy and framework', January 2018, https://www.england.nhs.uk/wp-content/uploads/2020/11/Revised-Never-Events-policy-and-framework-FINAL.pdf

11 NHS England, 'Provisional publication of Never Events reported as occurring between 1 April and 30 November 2021', 13 January 2022, https://www.england.nhs.uk/wp-content/uploads/2022/01/Provisional-publication-NE-1-April-30-November-2021.pdf

12 NHS England, 'Never Events data', https://www.england.nhs.uk/patient-safety/never-events-data/

13 CQC, 'Opening the door to change: NHS safety culture and the need for transformation', December 2018, https://www.cqc.org.uk/sites/default/files/20181224_openingthedoor_report.pdf

14 National Advisory Group on the Safety of Patients in England, 'Improving the safety of patients in England', August 2013, https://assets.publishing.service.gov.uk/government/uploads/system/uploads/attachment_data/file/226703/Berwick_Report.pdf

15 DHSC, 'High quality care for all: NHS Next Stage Review final report', 20 June 2008, https://www.gov.uk/government/publications/high-quality-care-for-all-nhs-next-stage-review-final-report

16 David Dalton, 'Leadership: values, mind-set and behaviours', King's Fund lecture, 2 October 2014, https://www.kingsfund.org.uk/sites/default/files/media/Leadership%20lecture%203%20-%202%20Oct.pdf

17 CQC, 'Salford Royal Hospital', https://www.cqc.org.uk/location/RM301

18 HCL, 'If the NHS was a country, how big would it be? Latvia, roughly', 23 February 2018, https://hclworkforce.com/blog/nhs-country-big-latvia-roughly/

Chapter 14: Zero

1 Mersey Care NHS Foundation Trust, 'No force first', https://www.merseycare.nhs.uk/health-and-wellbeing/what-recovery/no-force-first

2 Denis Campbell, 'Hunt urges NHS mental health units to prevent inpatient suicides', *Guardian*, 31 January 2018, https://www.theguardian.com/society/2018/jan/31/hunt-urges-nhs-mental-health-units-prevent-inpatient-suicide

3 Figures provided by Joe Rafferty.

4 ONS, 'Suicides in England and Wales: 2020 registrations', 7 September 2021, https://www.ons.gov.uk/peoplepopulationandcommunity/births deathsandmarriages/deaths/bulletins/suicidesintheunitedkingdom/ 2020registrations

5 Hayley Richardson, '"It was like someone threw a grenade in my house"', 11 August 2021, https://www.dailymail.co.uk/femail/article-9882995/ Father-student-killed-starting-Cambridge-says-wont-let-twice.html

6 ONS, 'Suicides in England and Wales'.

7 British Psychological Society, 'Understanding and preventing suicide: a psychological perspective', 11 September 2017, https://www.bps.org.uk/ sites/www.bps.org.uk/files/Policy/Policy%20-%20Files/Understanding %20and%20preventing%20suicide%20-%20a%20psychological%20 perspective.pdf

8 Zero Suicide Alliance, https://www.zerosuicidealliance.com

Chapter 15: Patient Power

1 Sally Davies, *Whose Health Is It, Anyway?* (Oxford: OUP, 2020), p. 7.

2 CQC, 'Care directory', https://www.cqc.org.uk/about-us/transparency/ using-cqc-data#directory

3 DHSC, Independent Medicines and Medical Devices Safety Review report, 8 July 2020, https://www.gov.uk/government/publications/ independent-medicines-and-medical-devices-safety-review-report

4 'Findings, Conclusions and Essential Actions from the Independent Review of Maternity Services at the Shrewsbury and Telford Hospital

NHS Trust', 30 March 2022, https://www.ockendenmaternityreview.org.uk/

5 WHO, 'Global patient safety action plan 2021–2030: towards eliminating avoidable harm in healthcare', 3 August 2021, https://apps.who.int/iris/rest/bitstreams/1360307/retrieve

6 WHO, 'WHO calls for urgent action to reduce patient harm in healthcare', 13 September 2019, https://www.who.int/news/item/13-09-2019-who-calls-for-urgent-action-to-reduce-patient-harm-in-healthcare and https://patientsafetymovement.org/patient-safety/the-facts/

INDEX

References to images are in *italics*.

Leabharlanna Poiblí Chathair Baile Átha Cli

Dublin City Public Libraries